M000216730

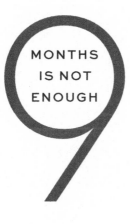
MONTHS
IS NOT
ENOUGH

9 MONTHS IS NOT ENOUGH

THE ULTIMATE PRE-PREGNANCY CHECKLIST TO CREATE A BABY-READY BODY AND BUILD GENERATIONAL HEALTH

ALEXANDRIA DEVITO, MS, CNS

LIONCREST
PUBLISHING

9 MONTHS IS NOT ENOUGH
The Ultimate Pre-Pregnancy Checklist to Create
a Baby-Ready Body and Build Generational Health
First Edition

ISBN   978-1-5445-4269-0   *Hardcover*
       978-1-5445-4267-6   *Paperback*
       978-1-5445-4268-3   *Ebook*

A book can change your life. This book can change your children's lives.

To future generations,

When we are sick, we focus inward—on healing ourselves.

When we are well, we focus outward— on contributing to the world.

This book is designed to give you the best starting shot at being vibrantly well—so that you can go forth and share your gifts with the world.

CONTENTS

FOREWORD

by Dr. Kara Fitzgerald, ND, IFMCP

I've been deep in the functional medicine space for my entire career, and along the way, I've had the pleasure of working with some extraordinarily talented clinicians. Alexandria DeVito is one of them.

Since becoming a doctor, my mission has been to reverse the global epidemic of chronic disease. I have built a thriving private practice in Connecticut, working with clinicians and patients around the world to provide personalized care through a functional medicine approach. My clinicians and I dig deep to get to the root cause of illness and support our patients in restoring vibrant health.

Through my work at the clinic, I began to focus on supporting healthy gene expression using a diet and lifestyle intervention that favorably influences DNA methylation. I was seeing remarkable results with my patients. Naturally, I wanted to take this a step further and create a research study to validate what we were seeing clinically. In 2021, I was fortunate to have the results of our pilot study published in the journal *Aging*. Our study showed that through adopting several lifestyle practices—such as eating a diet rich in specific nutrients, getting enough sleep, and practicing simple relaxation techniques—the participants were able to lower their biological age by an average of 3.23 years (compared to the control group, who received no intervention). This was huge!

Alexandria joined our clinical team as a functional nutritionist right around the time when I was first diving deeper into the topic of DNA methylation. She was on the front lines working with our patients to implement these diet and lifestyle interventions. You may be wondering what the heck DNA methylation has to do with preparing for pregnancy. Well, it turns out to be one of the most important pieces of the pre-pregnancy preparation puzzle. I think this explanation from my best-selling book *Younger You* does a nice job of walking us through why it's essential to take a more proactive approach to prepare from a genetic standpoint:

> What so few of us realize is that our genes themselves by and large do not dictate our fate. The truth is, while your DNA does provide the coding for everything that makes you who you are, its influence peaks at conception. Every day of your life since that initial meeting of sperm and egg, it's not what genes you have that matter. Of greater importance is which genes are turned on and which are turned off. And this you likely have a lot of control over...If you can nudge your genetic expression into tip-top shape, you'll be handing a pristine-as-possible imprint to your offspring. That's because your diet

and lifestyle choices affect the germ cells that you pass on to your children, which will, in turn, impact the germ cells that your children will pass on to their offspring (aka your grandchildren), and likely, generations beyond that, too.

How amazing is that! By preparing for pregnancy and improving our health, we can actually influence generational health. Talk about leaving behind an important legacy!

Now that I've piqued your interest, you're probably asking yourself, "Okay, how do I get my genetic expression into tip-top shape?" That is where this phenomenal book by Alexandria comes in.

Alexandria has laid out an easy-to-follow checklist to walk you through the process of preparing your body for conception. She has managed to distill a wealth of information into this comprehensive guide, information that has not been widely available until now. She has made this information approachable so that anyone can take steps to improve their epigenetic expression. In addition to writing this book, Alexandria also founded a company to make the solution, a functional medicine approach to pre-pregnancy preparation, widely accessible.

It was an honor to be asked to write this foreword for Alexandria. It's not lost on me how the timing of our journeys came together—when I was deep in DNA methylation and gene expression—and the lasting impact it has had on her work in the world. It's profound to see the ripple effects of our collective missions and how they build on one another to create a broader impact in the world. The information she is sharing in this book is essential for us to understand and enact on our pre-pregnancy journey. I cannot understate that fact: to reverse the infertility epidemic, which sits at the front of the chronic disease epidemic, we need to adopt these principles. By reading this book and following its guidance, you'll be making a huge difference in your health and the health of your future family.

THE FERTILITY GAP

What Doctors Aren't Telling You about Your Fertility

"Start taking a prenatal vitamin," her doctor said.

"Sounds good. What else can I be doing to increase my chances of getting pregnant?" Tihanna asked.

"That's about it for now. If you haven't been able to conceive after twelve months of trying, please come back to see me," her doctor continued.

"Okay. What about my husband? Is there anything that I should tell him to do to prepare?"

"Nope. Is there anything else that you want to discuss today?" the doctor said as she got up to walk out of the room.

"Ummm, no. I guess that's it for now," Tihanna said in disbelief.

That was the end of the conversation—a conversation Tihanna had waited six weeks for.

Let's rewind a bit. Tihanna is a thirty-three-year-old corporate lawyer. She is a successful but stretched working professional. She is highly efficient and organized but consistently has a long list of demands on her time. She and her husband have just decided that they would like to start trying to have kids in the next six months. Since Tihanna is a planner, she wanted to get a jump on things. She made an appointment with her ob-gyn to figure out the best next steps.

She wasn't sure if the fifteen years that she was on birth control might affect her ability to get pregnant. She originally went on the pill to help with acne; that hadn't been an issue for years, but she worried it might come back once she went off birth control and wasn't sure what to do if it did. She wondered whether her higher-than-average stress levels might affect her ability to get pregnant. She was also fairly health-conscious, watching her diet and exercising regularly, but she wasn't sure if she was in optimal health to support her goal of getting pregnant. Most of the time, she felt great, but she struggled with bloating and indigestion after meals and still got occasional urinary tract infections. She wondered whether those things could potentially affect her ability to conceive.

All of these questions lingered in her mind as she visited her ob-gyn to try to get some answers. She had already searched online for some perspective, but the data was all over the place—quite confusing and conflicting. Unfortunately, she didn't get the guidance she was looking for from her doctor either. Her doctor's response felt…inadequate.

She had an instinct that she could be doing more to prepare for pregnancy—much like she had prepared for everything else in her life (LSATs, law school, her wedding, etc.).

MAYBE YOU CAN RELATE?

You can't quite put your finger on it, but it's been on your mind, and you want to start doing *something* to support your fertility so your body is ready when you decide that it's time (whether that's three months from now or five years from now). You think you're healthy but wonder, *Am I really?* You're not alone.

WHY YOU'RE STRESSED ABOUT GETTING PREGNANT

I've interviewed and surveyed thousands of females like Tihanna about their fertility. When I ask whether they are anxious about their ability to get pregnant, the average answer I get is 7 (on a scale from 0–10, with 0 being cool as a cucumber and 10 being cold-sweat-level anxiety). This is true *regardless of* personal or family health history. In other words, women are anxious about their ability to get pregnant irrespective of whether they have known chronic health conditions that may interfere with their ability to get pregnant or whether they have any family history of infertility.

This is called reproductive anxiety. It's real—and it's on the rise. Reproductive anxiety is the feeling of stress that arises when you think about your fertility, including your ability to get pregnant, sustain a healthy pregnancy, or have a healthy baby.

Maybe it's because women are getting pregnant a bit later in life and have been told that this may make getting pregnant harder.

Maybe it's because many women have friends who have struggled with infertility and they've watched how taxing an experience it can be.

Maybe it's because there is so much fear-mongering out there around women's health in general that it's hard to figure out what to believe.

Maybe You're Worried Too?

You may be in a similar spot right now to Tihanna, looking around for reliable resources on fertility and feeling pretty frustrated…and simultaneously underwhelmed and overwhelmed by what you are finding. It's not your fault that you can't find what you are looking for. *There is a huge fertility gap.*

THE FERTILITY GAP

Dr. Sara Gottfried, a Harvard-trained gynecologist and bestselling author, who coined the term "fertility gap" said it best:

> When it comes to fertility, there are crucial facts that doctors don't share with you which are vital to your future childbearing. I call it the fertility gap. The fertility gap is largely unknown and unacknowledged in mainstream medicine, and few women have access to the secrets that could boost your fertility naturally.[1]

There are so many things that mainstream medicine and media aren't addressing when it comes to getting and staying pregnant. For example, have you ever been told any of the following?

- If you are having period problems, there is a higher probability that you will have trouble conceiving. Period problems, which can include irregular or absent periods, unusually heavy or long periods, irregular ovulation, or painful periods, are incredibly common, but they are definitely not normal (i.e., how your body was designed to operate). Period symptoms are indicator lights about what's going on in your body—and with your fertility.

- If you went on birth control for any reason besides pregnancy prevention (e.g., painful periods, acne, heavy bleeding), you likely had an underlying hormonal imbalance, and that hormonal imbalance can increase the timeline to get pregnant once you go off birth control. More than likely, that hormonal imbalance still exists but was masked by taking birth control. It can take up to a year to restore a regular period after going off birth control. And this restoration usually requires proactive remediation; unfortunately, you can't just cross your fingers and hope it will happen.

- Egg quality is modifiable *regardless of your age*, as long as you are still cycling. Despite the rhetoric that "age is the only predictor of fertility," not all thirty-year-olds or thirty-five-year-olds are created equally on a cellular level. The "life in your years" (biological age) matters more than the "years in your life" (chronological age). For example, just as smoking can negatively impact your egg quality, so can a poor diet, chronic stress, and environmental toxins—and all of these factors can be modified.

- **The healthier you are, the greater your chances of conceiving and carrying a child full term.** This may seem obvious, but if you have one or more chronic diseases (e.g., high blood pressure, diabetes, hypothyroidism), both you and your future baby will benefit from addressing them *before* you conceive.

Most women that I have spoken with have not been told any of these things. Neither was I. Despite this, I am here to tell you that there is so much that you can do to *get ready* to get pregnant. This pre-pregnancy preparation process is what this entire book is about. Throughout this book, I am going to expose the "fertility gap" that's keeping people in the dark when it comes to their reproductive ability. We are going to explore the different components of your health that may be indicative of imbalances in your body that can impact your fertility. Then, I am going to help you figure out specifically what to do about it to increase your chances of getting pregnant and having a healthy pregnancy and baby.

PRECONCEPTION IS THE NEW FERTILITY

Let's take a step back. How did I get here, and why should you even care about what I have to say on this topic?

I am a preconception expert, one of very few in the world. This is not the same thing as a fertility expert. I would argue

that fertility is a subset of preconception, but not the other way around. Fertility is focused on helping you to get pregnant—it's a binary outcome. Preconception is focused on helping you to get pregnant *and* have a healthy pregnancy and baby. We are missing the mark if you're able to get pregnant but can't sustain that pregnancy to term—or if that pregnancy leads to complications for you or your baby. Unfortunately, this is what we are seeing more and more often. Myopically focusing on getting pregnant is not enough; we need to set ourselves and our future babies up for success by making sure that our foundation is as solid as possible, leading to both easier conception and healthier babies.

I spent my early career in the corporate world—investment banking, management consulting, and an MBA from Harvard Business School. Then I transitioned to clinical practice. I went back to school to get my master's in nutrition as well as a certification as a functional medicine practitioner (one of only about two thousand in the world and only ~50 of which are also nutritionists, at the time of this writing). Then I started working as a clinical nutritionist focused on women's health.

What happened next surprised and disturbed me. I watched as clients ping-ponged between their doctor, their acupuncturist, their therapist, and me, all in search of clear guidance and direction on their fertility journey. I also watched heartbroken as friend after friend struggled to navigate the confusing and conflicting information out there about what to do when they were ready to conceive.

At some point, I couldn't ignore the repeated and remarkably consistent accounts from women across the country who shared similar stories about their provider encounters to what I described above with Tihanna. I finally realized that, unfortunately, many doctors are not trained in or equipped to provide adequate pre-pregnancy care. And it's not their fault! I have many close friends who are also doctors, and I have deep compassion for the challenges they face in providing sufficient care in the current medical system. Most doctors are trying to care for their patients in the best ways they can despite all the constraints that they operate with on a daily basis. Even if they wanted to engage more in pre-pregnancy care, in many cases, their hands are tied. They are operating in a system that is not designed or incentivized for this type of care. In fact, the medical establishment has diagnosis codes used by insurance companies that usually do not give the option of engaging with you prior to twelve months of struggling to conceive! This is bonkers, and it needs to change.

Until that time comes, I decided to do something about it—and to help you do the same. I couldn't believe that there weren't any resources to help couples *plan for pregnancy*— just like they plan for a wedding or a career. Even the process of buying a house has more support and guidance today than getting pregnant does! It's time for a fresh approach, and that's exactly what I'm going to be sharing with you. My goal is to normalize preconception preparation and make the process accessible to as many people as possible.

GET READY TO GET PREGNANT

When you're planning for a family, you want everything to go right. But you may have been told there's nothing that you can do—save for good genes and good luck. As a result, I find that people fall into one of two camps when it comes to getting pregnant: either they adopt a defeatist/laissez-faire attitude (there's not much I can do about it, so I'll just roll the dice and see what happens), or they adopt a militant approach (I have no idea what will work, so I will do all the things).

Instead of this binary equation where we either completely give up or go into maximum overdrive, I'd like to offer a different possibility. After working with hundreds of clients, running more lab tests than I can count, and poring over hundreds of peer-reviewed scientific studies and publications, I've discovered a better way to approach fertility proactively, and I can't wait to share it with you. I'll show you what factors are within your control based on the latest science. Spoiler alert: it involves more than taking a prenatal vitamin.

This proactive approach to fertility is the same one that we use at the company I founded. Poplin is the first pre-pregnancy wellness company. We help individuals and couples *get ready* to get pregnant. Poplin focuses on the *one* thing that I discovered that matters most when it comes to enhancing fertility and increasing the likelihood of having healthy children: pre-pregnancy preparation for both you and your reproductive partner.

Most people don't have access to work one-on-one with practitioners like me or to utilize assisted reproductive services. I wrote this book to give you, the reader, the knowledge and tools to arm yourself with the ability to take control of your own preconception journey—from wherever you live and whatever your starting point.

Please note: I will use the terms preconception and pre-pregnancy interchangeably throughout this book. They refer to the same time period.

ANCIENT PREGNANCY PREPARATION RITUALS

Did you know that most ancient cultures had pregnancy preparation rituals? These rituals usually included both partners. For example, according to *Deep Nutrition* by Catherine Shanahan, the Maasai tribes only allowed couples to marry after spending a few months drinking milk during the wet season, when rains led to lusher grass and, therefore, much more nutrient-dense milk. The entire tribe accommodated the newly married couple, who they presumed would get pregnant soon.[2] How cool is that?

WHY FOCUS ON PRE-PREGNANCY PREPARATION?

We focus so much time and energy on not being pregnant and then on being pregnant that we don't even consider the critical interim step: *getting pregnant*. Getting pregnant deserves a discussion unto itself—how to do it naturally (if you so choose), joyfully, and as gracefully as possible. This is the new science of preconception.

In fact, both the American College of Obstetricians and Gynecologists (ACOG) and the Centers for Disease Control (CDC) agree with the focus on preconception care. The

CDC found that the #1 way to enhance fertility and decrease the incidence of infertility is through better preconception care.[3] ACOG recommends pre-pregnancy counseling for *all women who want to become pregnant within the next year*.[4] When you plan and prepare for pregnancy *before* you want to get pregnant, it does two things:

1. It makes it easier to get pregnant.
2. It increases the likelihood of having a healthy baby.

PREPARE FOR PREGNANCY LIKE YOU WOULD FOR A WEDDING

If you've had a wedding (or even attended one), you know how much planning and care go into it. Most people spend at least a year planning for a wedding. The dress, the flowers, the music selection, the location, the attendee list. Every detail is thoughtfully crafted and executed. The attention to detail is exceptional.

I suggest that we consider applying this same level of attention, rigor, and forethought to our baby-making as we do to our wedding-making. Just like you prepare for your wedding months or even years in advance, the time it takes to set the stage for your baby is far in advance of conceiving. A growing body of research confirms that a bit of legwork upfront to prepare for your pregnancy can increase your chances of success down the road with a boost to your fertility and a higher likelihood of having a healthy pregnancy and baby.

It doesn't matter if this is your first or fifth pregnancy. It doesn't matter if you are twenty-three or forty-three. It doesn't matter if you are considered "low risk" or "high risk." *Everyone can benefit from pre-pregnancy preparation.*

That's exactly why we are here. This entire book is dedicated to the one thing that matters most when it comes to enhancing fertility and setting the stage for a healthy baby: preconception preparation (for both you and your reproductive partner). While the do-it-yourself (DIY) approach can be helpful for many things in life, sometimes big undertakings lend themselves to a professional helping hand. Just like a great wedding planner can help guide you through the process, this book can serve as your de facto "baby planner." I want to empower you to take the baby-making process into your own hands—and to help you short-circuit the process as much as possible based on my years of experience. This book was designed to remove the guesswork and guide you step-by-step through the process of preparing for pregnancy. If you're a planner like me, you're going to love it.

PUBLIC SERVICE ANNOUNCEMENT

For the male reproductive partners reading this book, first of all, kudos to you. Your future family appreciates your efforts. You may be wondering what your role is in this whole process. Dr. Michael Lu summarizes it well: "Sperm and support!" That's it. I mean, that's not really it, but in essence, it is. Your sperm carries your DNA that will be passed on to your future children. You want to pass on the best goods that you possibly can. The actions you take in the preconception period will be translated into the epigenetic material that sets the foundation for your child's lifelong health. This is literally your one shot to contribute your stuff. It's not a time to skimp. This entire book has recommendations for how to make that happen. In addition, this is an opportunity for you to demonstrate to your partner that you're all in. There is no greater support than doing the work yourself alongside your partner and taking mutual interest in and responsibility for the outcome. Most of all, I want you to know that your health and your participation really matter—you're an incredibly important part of this process, and I am so glad that you're here with us!

SO WHERE DO YOU START?

When people start trying to get pregnant these days, they often spend countless waking hours researching...and stressing...and then researching some more. Ultimately, in their pursuit of parenthood, they try to do all the things. But there are only a few things that you *actually* need to be doing to make your pregnancy dreams a reality. This is where this book comes in. I have identified how to simplify your efforts so you can focus exclusively on baby-making tasks and forget the rest of the noise out there. I did the legwork so you don't have to—though I know most of you are avid planners and researchers, so I would still encourage you to do your own digging and validating.

The approach found in this book, and amplified through Poplin, follows a scientifically backed method. No more trying to cobble together all the available resources out there in blogs and forums, grasping at straws to find out what is scientifically sound. I will share a comprehensive pre-pregnancy roadmap that synthesizes all the available information and tools into a one-stop shop for transforming your body, mind, and environment to optimize your fertility and improve your child's chances of lifelong health.

Much of what I will share is not widely discussed or understood in conventional circles, so I am here to get out the megaphone and share the goods with you. There are a lot of old wives' tales, unvalidated science, and general misinformation running around out there when it comes to reproductive health. My goal is to cut through the noise and bring you real talk. And, of course, to help you become a healthy mama or papa! The Poplin method is everything I was looking for to help my clients and my friends but couldn't find.

I believe that every female has the right to have choice and agency over her conception process—on her terms and on her timing. I believe that every female should have access to unbiased data to help her make the best decisions for herself and her family. And I believe that every male partner or donor should be welcomed into this journey and given the information and opportunity to participate too.

We are going to start rewriting this fertility dialogue together. Just by picking up this book, you've already taken steps in a positive direction. You've recognized that the current paradigm isn't working, and you've opened yourself up to another approach.

Please note: Though I just spent time telling you that I am a preconception expert and I endeavor to provide ample evidence to support the clinical points that I make throughout this book, I encourage you to read this book with an appropriate dose of skepticism. Don't just take my word for it. Read the book. Scour the references. Do your own digging. I aim to offer possibilities, not promises, of what can be available when you optimize the entire process of preparing to conceive. At every step of the way, I encourage you to be an active and informed participant in this journey. I will lay out the scientific rationale, and you get to decide what's best for you and your family.

IS THIS BOOK RELEVANT FOR ME?

If you've ever wondered:

- I think I'm healthy, but am I *really*?
- What can I do *now* to prepare my body for pregnancy later?
- How can I optimize my chances of getting pregnant and carrying a healthy baby to term?
- Should my partner be doing anything to prepare themselves?

I've got you covered!

This book is for you if any of the following apply:

- You are planning to get pregnant within the next year.
- You aren't sure when you want to conceive yet but are a planner and want to take control of your fertility and family planning.

- You are hoping to avoid the long and harrowing journey you've heard about from others who have struggled to conceive.
- You are currently undergoing or about to initiate egg freezing or assisted reproductive technologies (e.g., in vitro fertilization or intrauterine insemination) and would like to increase your chances of a successful outcome.
- You want your pregnancy experience to be as seamless as possible, both by conceiving easily and by optimizing your baby's health.
- You are pursuing a second, third, or sixth pregnancy and want to optimize your health after a previous pregnancy.
- You are a friend or family member who wants to support a loved one on their fertility journey.

WHAT YOU'LL GET FROM THIS BOOK

In the next sixteen chapters, I am going to deconstruct the biggest fertility myths out there. If you are like the hundreds of other women I've spoken to, most of what you have been told is total BS. In place of these myths, I will tell you how to:

- Run specific testing to identify any potential underlying health issues that may interfere with you or your partner's/donor's fertility.
- Partner with your doctor to get a full preconception visit before you even start trying.

- Detoxify from the exposures in your environment that could be harming your hormones and fertility (these are "fertility blockers").

- Boost your nutrition stores that will be used as the building blocks for every cell of your future baby's body (affectionately referred to as "fertility boosters").

- Select the best preconception supplementation regimen for you and your reproductive partner.

And more.

All these things can contribute to improving your egg health (and your reproductive partner's sperm health) *regardless* of your age. *This is the new science of reproductive anti-aging.* I will show you how lifestyle upgrades during critical time periods can pave the way for getting pregnant easily, having a healthy pregnancy and giving birth to a vibrant baby.

BABY-READINESS ASSESSMENT

Want to jump in right away? I recommend Poplin's qualitative baby-readiness assessment as an initial starting point. This assessment will give you a quick read on what factors can impact fertility and pregnancy and where you may need some extra TLC. Go to *quiz.getpoplin.com* to get started.

Please note: This book is intended to be a resource for any individual who desires to have children, regardless of gender identity, sexual orientation, or relationship construct. Where possible, I have made efforts to use sex assigned at birth rather than gender identity and to be inclusive of different relationship constructs (e.g., reproductive partner, donor/ partner). That being said, much of the language used in this book is heteronormative and/or gendered and focused on couples. I hope you can adapt this message to your specific context, when relevant, and still find this resource valuable in your preconception journey.

CHAPTER SUMMARY

- Reproductive anxiety is real, and it's rising. It comes from the delta between the level of importance of having children (high) and the level of control we've been told we have over our ability to have children (low). High-importance, low-control situations lead to extreme anxiety.

- There is a profound fertility gap—a gap in information about reproductive health that can help you enhance your ability to conceive and have healthy children.

- Pre-pregnancy preparation for both reproductive partners is the most effective intervention to enhance fertility and improve the chances of having a healthy baby.

PART 1

THE PROBLEM

Your Body Was Designed to Conceive, but the Modern Environment Was Not

In the past several years, there have been a proliferation of startups in the fertility space. Fertility is clearly a huge problem that's top of mind for many, and it's inspiring to see so much interest and energy being poured into supporting individuals on their family-building journeys.

Companies are trying to address the financing around infertility because it's exorbitantly expensive and there's very little access to care. Companies are trying to build community around those who are struggling with infertility because it can be a very isolating and challenging experience. Companies are trying to improve outcomes with each assisted reproductive technology round through technological advances and better data feedback loops.

These are all incredible, much-needed services. If you notice, though, they are all focused on *infertility, not fertility*.

In addition to providing these services to individuals who need them, I think we also need to be asking a different question: *why is infertility rising in the first place?*

We seem to be skipping over that fundamental question. In order to address a problem, you first have to understand it. The answer to this question may open up a whole new set of questions and possibilities, such as: *is there a way to address the problem before it becomes a problem?*

Let's start our journey by discussing what's really going on, which will set the stage for new solutions to emerge.

WAITING TO ADDRESS FERTILITY UNTIL IT BECOMES INFERTILITY IS WAY TOO LATE

The Current State of (In)fertility

nfertility currently affects about 19 percent of married American women between the ages of fifteen and forty-nine years, continues to increase, and shows no signs of abating.[1] Moreover, infertility is likely underreported because many people aren't getting the help that they need. It's pretty dismal, and it's getting worse. Infertility is starting to become more the rule than the exception.

Technically, infertility is defined as a couple that is unable to conceive after a year of concerted trying (or six months of trying if the woman is above the age of thirty-five). If a couple is deemed "infertile" (don't even get me started on the stigma associated with a label like this), their options to pursue parenthood are fairly limited:

- They can continue to try naturally.
- They can pursue assisted reproductive technologies (ART for short).
- They can adopt.

If they continue to try naturally, they are left to their own devices to scour message boards and cobble together the right combination of supplements, alternative remedies, and "best-kept secrets" that might work.

ART is a marvel of modern medicine, and it has been transformative in many ways. In particular, it has expanded the conception opportunity for people who were previously unable to have biological children, such as same-sex couples, individuals who have undergone chemotherapy, and couples who are sterile due to structural abnormalities. However, for the vast majority of couples, ART is being used prematurely because it's the only game in town. In fact, Dr. Sami David, a leading reproductive endocrinologist based in New York City, estimates that approximately 50 percent of IVF is unnecessary.[2] Wow. Even if it's a fraction of that number, that's still a whole lot of unnecessary procedures!

If a couple chooses to pursue ART, there are two main types: IUI (intrauterine insemination) and IVF (in vitro fertilization). Lots of acronyms! IUI is when sperm are collected, washed, and concentrated and then placed directly inside the uterus around the time of ovulation. The hope is that the sperm will have a shorter swim into the fallopian tube and will be able to fertilize a waiting egg, resulting in pregnancy. IVF is when an egg is removed from a female's ovaries and fertilized with sperm in a laboratory; the fertilized egg, now called an embryo, is then returned to the female's womb to grow and develop. Unfortunately, ART is inaccessible for most people; in fact, according to the CDC, only about 3–7 percent of women utilize IUI or IVF services due to both cost and logistics issues.[3]

Even for the couples that do have access and choose to pursue ART, most are not prepared for the physical, emotional, and financial toll that infertility services can take. IVF involves daily injections and potent hormonal medications—it's intense. Because of this, females struggling with infertility report similar levels of anxiety and depression as those with cancer.[4] Infertility carries a heavy emotional load.

Beyond this, the average cost for a single IVF cycle is $23,050.[5] And 70 percent of IVF cycles fail.[6] Let that sink in for a minute. This means that couples have to try over and over again because the process is fairly ineffective. On average, according to FertilityIQ, couples go through more than two cycles to conceive a baby, costing $40,000 to $60,000.[7] Since most fertility treatments are not covered by insurance, couples are left to fend for themselves to pay for these services. Some employer-sponsored health plans offer fertility coverage, but those are few and far between.

You may wonder how couples are managing to pay for these exorbitant costs. According to Modern State of Fertility 2020:

- 77 percent are dipping into their savings accounts or 401(k)s.

- 60 percent are putting it on their credit cards or taking out personal loans.
- 26 percent are asking for help from their families.[8]

This is simply unsustainable.

There is also some new data suggesting that there are long-term implications for the babies conceived through ART (such as increased risk of pediatric cancers, autism, and intellectual impairment).[9] It's not yet clear whether it's the ART drugs and procedures themselves that increase these risks or whether these risks were already present and contributed to infertility in the first place—or possibly both.

WE NEED A BETTER WAY

Today, most of the time that we talk about fertility, it's in the context of infertility. As a society, we only address fertility once it becomes infertility, and that's *way too late*. Even for individuals who don't struggle with infertility, the path to getting pregnant is often overwhelming, confusing, and anxiety-provoking. *We need a better way*.

Unsurprisingly, because of all of the harrowing stories and statistics as outlined above, women want to do everything they can to avoid infertility. In fact, according to Modern State of Fertility 2020:

- 32 percent of women would rather give up vacations for ten years than experience infertility.
- 58 percent would rather break a bone.
- 30 percent would rather lose half their savings.[10]

Women are so scared of infertility that they would rather give up recreation for ten years, break a part of their body, or give up their financial security to avoid it altogether. Those numbers are staggering! *We need a better way.* The existing infertility solutions are woefully inadequate. They are broken, outdated, and insufficient. Most people don't have access to them. For those who do, they are physically, emotionally, and financially draining to an unconscionable degree. *We need a better way.*

Chronic childhood disease is on the rise—asthma, allergies, autism, diabetes, and ADHD, in particular. Today, 54 percent of children suffer from a chronic health condition.[11] This has increased dramatically in the last fifty to sixty years (from 2 percent in the 1960s). This is heartbreaking. *We need a better way.*

Here's a sneak peek of what's to come: There is now evidence to suggest that sowing the seeds for children's health starts far in advance of conception and continues through the first few years of life. The central idea in this book is that healthier parents conceive more easily and give birth to healthier babies. Building generational health starts with you—and it starts *before* you conceive. *This is a better way.*

CHAPTER SUMMARY

- The current infertility-centric model is broken. Infertility continues to rise, and current solutions are woefully inadequate: inaccessible for most, and financially, emotionally, and physically draining for the few who can access them.

- We need a better way. That better way involves focusing on the health of both reproductive partners before they conceive. Healthier parents conceive more easily and give birth to healthier babies.

2

EVERYTHING YOU'VE BEEN TOLD ABOUT FERTILITY IS WRONG

nspired by my mission to figure out how to help my clients and friends on their fertility journeys, I decided to do a deep dive on reproductive health. I pored over scientific studies. I evaluated case studies. I scoured lab tests. I read every book that I could find on the topic. What I found completely shocked me.

I thought I was a fairly educated and aware person, but *oh my goodness*, I realized that there was so much that I didn't know about my own damn body.

As a young girl, I was told that I could get pregnant any time of the month. That I was so fertile that if a guy even looked at me suggestively, he could impregnate me. As a woman in her thirties, I've now discovered that's totally not true. You are only fertile six days each month. I understand why I received that message as a teenager, but seriously, WTF?!

I was told that period symptoms were normal—bloating, breast tenderness, constant cramps. Lies. All lies. While period symptoms are *common*, they are definitely not *normal* (i.e., how your body was designed to operate). In fact, period symptoms are indicators of what's going on underneath the surface. For example, breast tenderness often indicates excess estrogen, and spotting can indicate low progesterone. *Who would've thought?*

I was also told that birth control is a panacea for all the things—it will empower you to go live your life as you deem fit; it will free you from the chains of an unpredictable period. And it did do those things. But it also had some nasty side effects. For me and for many of my clients, birth control became "birth control" by tanking libido. *Who needs to worry about getting pregnant if you never want to have sex in the first place?* I mean, come on!

I could go on and on, but you get the point. Needless to say, I was shocked and humbled.

I finally realized what was going on: *pretty much everything we have been told about our reproductive health and fertility is incomplete or flat-out wrong.*

I was incensed. Other women need to know this information too—not only about periods but about hormonal health and fertility in general.

UNLEARNING PRECEDES LEARNING

So much of what I learned about women's health and fertility through my clinical research and experience required me to *unlearn* what I was taught growing up and to relearn a new paradigm for functioning in the world.

Have you ever considered how much of life is "unlearning"? In many cases, unlearning precedes learning. You have to be able to let go of old beliefs and patterns first. Only then can you embrace new perspectives and skills.

Many of us have been taught what to believe by well-meaning doctors and the media. In some cases, this information has served us well. In other cases, not so much. The amount of information coming at us on a daily basis requires us to be diligent about what information we let in and allow to shape our lives.

In order to live consciously and deliberately, you have to be willing to question and critically evaluate whether the prevailing narrative still resonates with you. *Does this make logical sense? Is this consistent with my experience? Does this serve my interests?* And so on.

Much of what I now share with you will require a similar unlearning. It can be unsettling and liberating at the same time.

Ask yourself: *Am I open to the process of unlearning?* Growth often starts there.

In that spirit, let's talk about the biggest myths in fertility.

TOP FERTILITY MYTHS

MYTH #1: *Fertility rapidly declines after age thirty-five.*

TRUTH #1: *Fertility does decline with age, but it is not the precipitous drop you are led to believe it is.*

Many women have been taught that age is the only determinant of fertility and, in particular, that fertility rapidly declines after thirty-five. The storyline goes: once you turn thirty-five, you turn into a pumpkin—too bad, so sad for you; your egg count falls off a cliff, and there is nothing more you can do. Not only is this disempowering, but it's simply not true. The data does not support this conclusion.

The most commonly cited statistic to support this claim is that one out of three women over the age of thirty-five will fail to conceive after a year of trying. Here's the thing: the data for this conclusion comes from 1789 birth records. Talk about outdated! It was first cited in a paper published by Henri Leridon in the *Human Reproduction* journal, referencing birth records from eighteenth-century France; this would have been at a time before the availability of things like antibiotics and birth control pills, never mind reliable nutrition and healthcare access.[1] Women at that time likely were not even trying to conceive in their thirties and forties; in fact, they may have been actively trying to avoid it by having less sex or not having sex.

Rather than relying on two-centuries-old data, let's look at more recent studies. A 2004 publication by David Dunson looked at 780 healthy European couples actively and naturally trying to get pregnant across every age bracket. The results: of women aged twenty-seven to thirty-four years old, 86 percent of them conceived within one year of trying. Of women aged thirty-five to thirty-nine years old, 82 percent of them conceived within one year of trying. *That's only a 4 percent difference!*[2] Other more recent studies have found similar results. Likely, fertility does decline with age, but it is not the precipitous drop women are led to believe it is.

Moreover, the premise that egg quantity is the be-all and end-all of fertility is also faulty. For 95 percent of women, egg quantity is essentially irrelevant when it comes to getting pregnant. Let me say that again—for 95 percent of women, egg quantity is essentially irrelevant when it comes to getting pregnant. Premature ovarian failure only affects 1 percent of women, and diminished ovarian reserve affects about 5 percent of women under the age of thirty-five.[3] In fact, at age forty, the average woman still has over ten thousand eggs left.[4] This means that at every age, egg quality is more important than egg quantity. Rebecca Fett summarizes it well in her book *It Starts With the Egg*:

> The scientific research shows that egg quality is the single most important factor in determining whether an egg will fertilize and survive to the blastocyst stage. It also determines whether an embryo is capable of implanting and leading to a viable pregnancy.[5]

This myth assumes that all thirty-five-year-olds are created equal, which is simply not biologically true. Fertility is *not* solely dependent on age. There are many other factors that affect fertility besides age (and the good news is that unlike age, most of these factors are within your control). Which brings us to our next myth.

MYTH #2: *Age is the only predictor of fertility. There is nothing you can do to improve your fertility or affect the quality of your eggs.*

TRUTH #2: *As long as you are still cycling, you can improve the quality of your eggs. Age is only one factor of many that can affect your fertility.*

An extension of the myth above, because women are taught that age is the only predictor of fertility, they are also led to believe that there is nothing that they can do to improve their fertility—except maybe "age backward." I call bullshit on this one too. There are *tons* of things that you can do to improve your fertility. Your fertility is a barometer of your health. The healthier you are, the more fertile you are.

The biggest misunderstanding in fertility today is that your biological age is the same as your chronological age. In fact, for most people, their chronological age (actual age in years) is different from their biological age (the vibrancy and vitality of their cells and organs). It's like the difference between the "life in your years" and the "years in your life." I am sure you have seen this disparity in everyday life—people in their fifties who look like they are in their thirties and people in their thirties who look decades older. Clearly, we can see that people age at different rates, and it's probably not surprising that people with "harder" lifestyles (e.g., smoking, sleep deprivation, high stress) tend to age more quickly than those with "gentler" lifestyles (e.g., organic vegetable gardens, meditation circles). How you take care of yourself matters.

It is true that youth forgives a lot of ills. I'm guessing you've experienced this firsthand. When you were younger, you could bounce back from injuries, hangovers, and lack of sleep more quickly. Your body could weather more wear and tear. When you are young, your body is able to repair itself quickly and efficiently. As you get older, however, the repair process is less efficient and effective.

As we age, our arteries may become stiffer. Our bones may become less dense, and our muscles may lose strength. While these things are a function of age, they are not only a function of age; *they are also a function of health*. And your lifestyle is the biggest determinant of health. Because of this, people age at vastly different rates depending on how they live their day-to-day lives. For example, in the Blue Zones, the areas with the most concentrated number of centenarians in the world, people tend to live longer, happier, and healthier lives than their counterparts in other parts of the world. This isn't just a coincidence; it has been attributed to a set of nine healthy living principles, such as moving often, being part of a community, and eating a plant-rich diet.[6] I point this out because people assume that aging is linear and out of their control. But empirical and scientific evidence suggests otherwise.

In fact, certain scientists have found a way to calculate the difference between your chronological and biological age. To estimate biological age, you can look at certain health biomarkers such as blood pressure, blood glucose, liver function, maximal oxygen consumption, and cognitive ability to assess health status. Biological age is often a better measure of a person's health than chronological age; moreover, risk of certain age-related diseases, such as Alzheimer's, can be more closely associated with biological age than chronological age.[7]

The reason I bring all of this up is because age has been such a hot-button issue in fertility. Not all thirty-five-year-old women are biologically equal, though they are often treated as such by modern medicine. It would be shortsighted to use a person's chronological age alone to determine their health status. Yes, it is one piece of the puzzle, but it's not the whole puzzle by any means. Instead, your biological age is a much better predictor of health status... and, I would also suggest, fertility status.

At the risk of repeating myself again, age is one factor of many when it comes to fertility. Luckily, there are many other factors that you can control—diet, movement, sleep, stress management, and so on. Anything that you can do to improve your health also improves your fertility. Rather than overfocusing on your biological clock, recognize that you have so much more agency over your fertility than you have been led to believe and start making changes today to adopt a fertility-friendly lifestyle. That's exactly what this book is here to help you do.

The bottom line is that the older you are, the more your health matters when it comes to fertility. Regardless of age, there are specific steps that you can take to improve your egg health and uterine environment...and therefore, your fertility. (This is, of course, also true of males and sperm health.)

MYTH #3: You are a walking baby magnet. You ooze fertility. Getting pregnant is super easy. You don't have to do anything to prepare.

TRUTH #3: Getting pregnant is getting harder. Unlike your parents and grandparents, you likely need to prepare.

As kids, many of us were taught that getting pregnant is super easy. Middle school sexual education is designed to instill fear that pregnancy can happen at any second. As young adults, we hear the same message in the media. It's the storyline of every romantic comedy. One-night stand, got pregnant, fell in love. Happily ever after. The end.

Unfortunately, in the real world, it's not quite that simple, and that messaging is not helpful when you're in your twenties, thirties, or forties and actively trying to conceive. Despite what we may have been told as preteens, you cannot get pregnant at any time. There is a specific time period each month that you are fertile; you want to optimize for that time period if you are trying to get pregnant and stay away from that time period if you are trying to avoid pregnancy. In fact, there are only around six days each month that a female can get pregnant—the five days prior to ovulation and the day of ovulation itself. This is the so-called fertile window. Yeah, that was a huge eye-opener for me too. If you have sex outside this window (too early or too late), you will not be able to get pregnant that month. You want to be having sex *before* ovulation, so the sperm are raring and ready to go, waiting to fertilize the egg as soon as it's released from the follicle. That's why identifying this fertile window is a key part of getting pregnant seamlessly.

Moreover, even if you nail the timing piece of the equation, you also need a good egg, good sperm, and a welcoming environment for a successful conception. We will talk about that next.

MYTH #4: *Getting pregnant is a mythical, magical process, and you have no control over it.*

TRUTH #4: *There is a basic formula to getting pregnant.*

I put these myths back to back because they are a bit paradoxical—and I find that many people simultaneously believe both. Getting pregnant will be easy—and there's nothing I can do to control it.

To get pregnant, you need four things: Good egg + good sperm + proper timing + optimal environment (read: uterus)

You need a high-quality egg. Among other things, this means that it has high-functioning mitochondria. The pre-pregnancy checklist in Part 3 is all about improving egg quality through diet and lifestyle interventions.

You need a high-quality sperm. This means that it has proper motility and morphology. It also has high-functioning mitochondria. The pre-pregnancy checklist in Part 3 is all about improving sperm quality.

You need to have sex within your fertile window (which, as we discussed above, is five days prior to ovulation and the day of ovulation itself). See Chapter 16 for details on confirming ovulation and identifying your fertile window.

You need an optimal uterine environment. This includes good blood flow and minimal obstructions (e.g., fibroids). Many of the interventions in this book are also designed to improve endometrial receptivity. (In some cases, you may need medical intervention if there are significant structural abnormalities.)

MYTH #5: Hormonal birth control has no near-term impact on your fertility. All you have to do is stop the pill/ patch/injections, and your body will be ready to conceive.

TRUTH #5: Hormonal birth control can impair your time to conception if you do not take proactive steps to offset its effects.

Before we dive in, let me say this: for many reasons, birth control is intimately linked to women's rights, women's liberation, and women's advocacy. Birth control has given many women freedom, flexibility, and choice. In many ways, birth control has been an enabler of women's forward progress. For that, I hold reverence, and I am personally deeply grateful for the freedoms it offered me in my own life and career. But as with most things, there are two sides of the coin. In the case of birth control, we have spent so much time focusing on its accolades that we haven't left space for its downsides. As with *any* medication, there are side effects. Until recently, no one really cared about or talked about the side effects of hormonal birth control (e.g., pill, ring, shot, hormonal IUD). The benefits seemed to outweigh the costs. Now that we have more data on the costs, it might be time for a reevaluation. This is an incredibly personal decision, so I will share the data and let you decide what's best for you and your future family.

First, let's briefly cover how hormonal birth control works. Pills provide varying doses of synthetic estrogen and/or progesterone to suppress the body's natural rhythm of hormone secretion, prevent ovulation, and induce menstrual bleeding on a regular basis when inactive pills are taken. Essentially, they mimic the hormonal state of pregnancy. The withdrawal bleeding that takes place is not truly a period. Your hormones *do not* cycle as they regularly would, with estrogen rising in the first half of your cycle, follicle-stimulating hormone (FSH) stimulating follicle growth, luteinizing hormone (LH) initiating ovulation, and progesterone rising after ovulation.

Now that we understand how birth control operates, let's discuss its potential side effects and how some of these side effects may play a role in fertility challenges:

*Hormonal Birth Control Depletes the Body of
Key Nutrients, Many of which Are Critical for
Initiating and Maintaining Pregnancy*

The World Health Organization (WHO) has acknowledged for years that birth control pills can disrupt nutrient balance in the body. As far back as 1975, they were reporting that "oral contraceptives, which are now so widely used, have far-reaching metabolic effects on many tissues and organs, and these include effects on the levels and possibly the activities of various vitamins."[8] Specifically, studies have demonstrated key nutrient depletions occur in folic acid, vitamins B2, B6, B12, vitamin C, and vitamin E, as well as in the minerals magnesium, selenium, and zinc in women using birth control pills.[9] Because of this, most investigators recommend that supplemental vitamins like B2 and B6 be given to women on birth control pills, as well as B12 and vitamin C if they are deficient. Practically, I imagine one would be hard-pressed to find a doctor who routinely tested these vitamin levels when prescribing birth control pills or who counseled a patient about the need for supplementation. Many of these nutrients are critical for maintaining and sustaining a pregnancy and need to be replete prior to conception; otherwise, it will simply be harder to get and stay pregnant.

Hormonal Birth Control Can Alter the Gut Microbiome

Birth control can lead to a host of gut challenges, including leaky gut, yeast overgrowth, lack of microbial diversity, and issues with digestion and gut motility.[10] An altered microbiome can be responsible for a number of symptoms, including headaches, yeast infections, lowered immunity, and even mood disorders. In addition, a dysbiotic gut can also be transferred to your baby, predisposing them to things like asthma and allergies. The microbiome is also intimately linked to our immune function; a compromised microbiome can also lead to a compromised immune system, which can impact both fertility and pregnancy.[11]

Hormonal Birth Control Can Impair Detoxification,
Allowing a Toxic Hormonal Soup to Build Up in Your Body

Any time that hormones are imbalanced (too much or too little), fertility problems ensue. Excess estrogen, for example, is linked to fibroids, endometriosis, and even some cancers. I go into much more detail on the importance of proper detoxification for hormonal balance and fertility in Chapter 9, but I wanted to mention it here so you are aware of the potential impact of birth control on detoxification capacity.

Hormonal Birth Control Can Mask
Underlying Hormonal Imbalances

As I mentioned earlier, you do not actually get a period each month while on hormonal birth control; what seems like a period is a chemically induced "withdrawal bleed." Practically speaking, this means that your hormones don't fluctuate normally and naturally; therefore, your body does not produce many of the signs of hormonal dysfunction (e.g., acne, spotting, absent periods) that it otherwise would. Your body's symptom cascade is "silenced."

Here's the thing: 58 percent of women use oral contraceptive pills for reasons other than contraception.[12] These include indications like heavy menstrual bleeding, endo-metriosis, premenstrual syndrome (PMS), menstrual cycle regulation from things like polycystic ovary syndrome (PCOS) or amenorrhea (no period), and acne treatment. Many of these indications reflect a possible underlying hormonal imbalance to begin with.

This is where things get interesting: birth control pills are seductive because they are quite good at their job of creating the *appearance* of a regular menstrual cycle. Menstrual bleeding may lighten. Cramps may abate. Acne may resolve. Birth control is great at managing the *symptoms* of irregular cycles.

However, it is very important to understand that birth control does *nothing* to correct the underlying problem—the hormonal dysregulation that led to the menstrual symptoms in the first place. In effect, birth control pills are a Band-Aid; they cover up the problem, but they don't fundamentally fix it.

If you went on hormonal birth control for *any reason other than contraception*, such as heavy periods, severe cramps, or acne, then you likely had an underlying hormone imbalance causing those symptoms, and it is likely to still be present once you discontinue hormonal birth control.

If you developed an underlying hormone imbalance while on birth control from changes like weight gain or loss, new life stressors, medication, or an endocrine or autoimmune disorder, the imbalance may go undetected for years.

In addition, birth control plays a role in elevating thyroid-binding globulin (TBG), sex hormone binding globulin (SHBG), and corticosteroid-binding globulin (CBG).[13]

Effectively, this means that it inactivates many of your hormones and makes your reproductive and endocrine system work harder.

Given the convenience and effectiveness they afford women, many remain on birth control pills for years at a time and don't realize that they have hormonal problems until they go off hormonal birth control and try to get pregnant. Hormonal birth control has covered up the underlying issue. When a woman's regular cycles do not immediately resume, it can take a lot of time and backtracking to identify and correct the hormonal issue that lay hidden for so long.

Sometimes, these underlying hormonal issues have been festering for years; in many cases, the symptoms of these underlying issues were the initial reason the woman went on birth control. Again, the important thing to understand is that birth control didn't solve the underlying problem (which was an imbalance of hormones); it only masked the problem by quieting the symptoms. When you come off birth control, you are still left with that underlying problem, which definitely didn't get resolved and may have even progressed. *Pretty frustrating, huh?*

Hormonal Birth Control Can Cause Post-Pill Amenorrhea

Hormonal birth control essentially shuts down the communication system between your brain and your ovaries. This means that it might take a bit of time for your brain to get the message to reinitiate regular cycling and ovulation after having been "turned off." Because of this, many women experience "post-pill amenorrhea," which is irregular or absent periods once they go off birth control. It can take some time for your cycle to normalize again. This time period varies widely but can take up to twelve months.

This isn't about birth control being good or bad. As with any medication, it's about weighing the benefits and risks. And it's about your unique situation and priorities. It's just important to be an informed consumer, and you can't be informed if no one gives you all the facts.

The big takeaway here is that birth control can mask underlying hormonal imbalances while you are on it. Even once you're off it, the effects of hormonal birth control can increase barriers and therefore time to getting pregnant through nutrient deficiencies, altered microbiome function, and impaired detoxification. It often takes concerted compensatory actions and adequate time to transition off birth control and ensure that your hormonal system is in good shape before trying to conceive.

MYTH #6: The burden and responsibility of getting pregnant falls on the female reproductive partner.

TRUTH #6: Biology does not care about the cultural construct that fertility is a female problem. Getting pregnant is a couple's issue.

I'm going to keep this short and to the point.

Did you know that sperm counts have dropped 60 percent in the last forty years globally?[14]

Did you know that 30 percent of all infertility cases are related to male factors?[15]

Did you know that poor sperm quality can increase miscarriage risk?[16]

Did you know that sperm quality can also affect autism risk?[17]

Needless to say, a male reproductive partner's contribution is critical to your ability to get pregnant, have a healthy pregnancy, and have a healthy baby. Your partner (or donor) is literally 50 percent of the equation when it comes to your future baby.

It takes two healthy individuals to create the raw materials necessary to make a baby. Lucky for us, the same things that improve egg quality also improve sperm quality. If you are going to be conceiving together, you might as well start preparing together too.

MYTH #7: *Infertility is the same thing as sterility.*

TRUTH #7: **Infertility is not the same thing as sterility.**

Let's start with some definitions:

If you are infertile, you are unable to conceive within a year of unprotected intercourse.

If you are sterile, you are physiologically incapable of conceiving.

Infertility is about historical performance rather than capacity. To oversimplify, infertility is reversible; sterility is not.

One study estimated that sterility occurred in about 1 percent of the female population.[18] Sterility status does not change with age. Sterility can occur as a result of congenital malformations of the uterus or testes, surgical procedures or chemotherapy treatments, for example. Unfortunately, if you are sterile, you can't change that fact, but you can still pursue parenthood by exploring alternative reproductive techniques or adoption.

In that same study, infertility was estimated at 8 percent for women aged nineteen to twenty-six years, 13–14 percent for women aged twenty-seven to thirty-four years, and 18 percent for women aged thirty-five to thirty-nine years (again, we only see a 4 percent difference in fertility rates between women aged twenty-seven to thirty-four and women aged thirty-five to thirty-nine).[19] Infertility rates rise with age, mostly correlated with egg quality and overall health. The researchers concluded that "increased infertility in older couples is attributable primarily to declines in fertility rates rather than to absolute sterility. Many infertile couples will conceive if they try for an additional year."[20]

What do we make of this? Older couples may take longer to conceive than younger couples. This may be because older couples are having sex less frequently than younger couples. It may also be because older couples are less healthy than younger couples, which may complicate their pregnancy attempts. There are many factors at play.

The point here is that only a *very, very, very* small percentage of the population cannot conceive at all—far smaller than we've been led to believe.

Let's go a bit deeper.

Infertility is a medical diagnosis. As mentioned above, it literally just means that you are unable to conceive after a year of concerted trying (or six months if you're over the age of thirty-five). One year is a fairly arbitrary cutoff.

Our language really matters here. There are a number of medical terms that need a rebrand, and *infertility* is one of them. ("Incompetent uterus" and "advanced maternal age" are also at the top of the list!) When you put "in" at the front of a word, it implies "not." For example, *inconsistent* means *not* consistent, *inconclusive* means *not* conclusive, *inconsiderate* means *not* considerate. It naturally follows that infertility means *not* fertile. Yet that's not biologically correct.

Let's break this down.

Fertile = capable of reproducing

Infertile = *not* capable of reproducing

This is a misnomer because fertility is a spectrum, not a binary on/off switch.

As mentioned above, only a small percentage of people are not capable of reproducing on their own. In my experience, most people diagnosed with "infertility" are actually experiencing impaired fecundity (or subfertility). Impaired fecundity refers to individuals who have difficulty getting pregnant or carrying a pregnancy to term—due to a constellation of factors that dampen natural fertility. This does not mean that you are not able to conceive; it means that you are not able to conceive right now—the key is to figure out *why*. When you identify the fertility blockers and remove those interlopers, the body is often able to conceive naturally.

MYTH #8: You froze your eggs, so you're good to go.

TRUTH #8: Egg freezing is still a fairly new
procedure, and it is not foolproof.

Kudos to you—you were proactive and you did what you thought you needed to do in order to protect your fertility. I hate to be the bearer of bad news on this one, especially as a type-A planner myself, but egg freezing is, at best, a backup plan.

I recently had a conversation with a woman who froze her eggs in her thirties like the forward-thinking planner that she was. When she went to use them a decade later, they didn't take. Not after round one of IVF. Not after round two of IVF. Future rounds weren't looking much better. She told me she would have made different decisions if she had known this was even a possibility.

I want you to know.

First, ART success rates are significantly higher with fresh eggs than with frozen eggs. In fact, a recent study found that the percentage of individuals who ultimately had a baby after undergoing egg freezing and subsequently using their frozen eggs was just 39 percent.[21] Second, egg quality matters at the time of egg freezing—and it's often not enough to just rely on age. Age is one factor of many that influences egg quality. As we discussed earlier in this chapter, your biological age is not the same thing as your chronological age. Because of this, you can prepare for egg freezing in the same way that you'd prepare to get pregnant.

MYTH #9: You can just start trying to conceive
and if that doesn't work, you can pursue IVF.

TRUTH #9: Waiting until you have an issue
conceiving makes getting pregnant harder, more
expensive, and more emotionally taxing to address.

IVF is not foolproof. In fact, IVF is far less effective than the mainstream narrative would have us believe. According to the CDC, it fails 70 percent of the time, forcing most individuals to undergo multiple rounds in their pursuit of parenthood.[22] It is also incredibly invasive and expensive at an average per-cycle price of $23,050 for drug and treatment costs.[23] Given that most individuals pay out of pocket for these fertility costs, IVF is best used as a last resort rather than a first line of defense. There are many alternatives that are less invasive and less expensive that can be pursued prior to IVF. Regardless, planning and preparing for pregnancy in advance makes it easier to get pregnant whether that's naturally or with ART.

MYTH #10: If you've struggled to conceive, you'll require medical procedures to get pregnant.

TRUTH #10: For the vast majority of the population, addressing modifiable lifestyle factors is enough to achieve successful conception, even if you have previously struggled.

It's natural to think this since all the solutions to infertility problems are "medical" in nature. However, getting pregnant is usually *not* a medical issue—it often involves lifestyle and environmental components. Remember, only 1 percent of the population is sterile.

I know this because I have personally seen so many couples conceive naturally after they have been deemed "infertile" by the traditional medical establishment. They utilized dietary, lifestyle, supplementation, and, when necessary, medication interventions to improve their preconception health.

It's pretty miraculous. As Christa Orecchio, functional nutritionist, says, "Give the body what it needs, take away what it doesn't, and the body will heal itself."

Usually, unexplained infertility just means *not yet explained* infertility. If you do the type of broad screening suggested in Chapter 6, often you can get to the root cause of infertility. Once you find the root cause, the vast majority of infertility is modifiable, often through diet and lifestyle; occasionally, medications and procedures are needed—but that's the exception, not the rule.

With all these myths running around, it's surprising that anyone gets knocked up these days. But seriously, the next time someone tells you something disempowering about your health or your ability to get pregnant, question it.

In fact, one more thing before you go: did you know that new animal research is suggesting we may be able to create new eggs from stem cells?[24] This flies in the face of the idea that women are born with all the eggs they will ever have. It suggests that despite popular belief to the contrary, a woman's ovarian reserve is not fixed at birth; her ovarian reserve does indeed have the capacity for regeneration.

Why am I telling you this? Because it underscores the point I've been making this entire chapter: we have to question *everything* we have been told about our fertility. Advice circulating in doctors' offices and fertility clinics is simply not keeping pace with the latest research. Science is evolving, and we should evolve with it. Blindly following outdated medical models is unwise at best and unsafe at worst. Whether this scientific development turns out to be valid or not, the point remains: when it comes to your health, keep an open mind, question things constantly, and be flexible enough to incorporate new information into your operating model as you go.

CHAPTER SUMMARY

- Everything you've been told about getting pregnant is wrong. Most people's sexual education occurred at age thirteen. What was fit for purpose at age thirteen (presumably to avoid pregnancy) is not fit for purpose in your twenties, thirties, and forties (if you want to pursue pregnancy).

- Fertility does decline with age, but it is not the precipitous drop that women are led to believe it is.

- As long as you are still cycling, you can improve the quality of your eggs. Your biological age, *not* your chronological age, is the biggest risk factor for all chronic disease, including infertility risk.

- Getting pregnant is getting harder. Unlike our parents and grandparents, we need to prepare.

- There is a basic formula for getting pregnant: good egg + good sperm + proper timing + optimal environment (read: uterus)

- Hormonal birth control can impair your time to conception if you do not take proactive steps to offset its effects (depleting the body of key nutrients, altering gut microbiome, impairing detoxification, masking underlying hormonal imbalances, and/or causing post-pill amenorrhea).

- Biology does not care about our social construct that fertility is a female problem. It is a 50/50 biological equation between female reproductive partner and male reproductive partner.

- Infertility is not the same thing as sterility. We are experiencing an epidemic of subfertility (impaired ability to conceive) rather than infertility (inability to conceive). Infertility is a medical diagnosis based simply on time to conception, not a specified underlying medical condition, and it's a complete misnomer. Ninety-nine percent of the population has the capacity to conceive physiologically (though there may be other reasons for medical intervention, as in same-sex couples).

- Egg freezing is not foolproof.

- IVF is not foolproof.

- Even if you've struggled to conceive, addressing modifiable lifestyle factors can often lead to successful conception (with or without additional medical intervention).

3

WHY GETTING PREGNANT IS HARDER TODAY THAN FOR PREVIOUS GENERATIONS

Now that we've busted some fertility myths, let's talk about what's really going on here.

As we discussed in the previous chapter, most women are taught that getting pregnant is easy-peasy. Our bodies were designed for this, weren't they?

TLDR: Yes, our bodies were designed for this, but our modern lifestyle and environment were not.

We are seeing a decline in the fertility of both males and females. As Shanna Swan, the author of *Count Down*, notes, "In some parts of the world, the average twentysomething woman today is less fertile than her grandmother was at thirty-five."[1] Sperm counts are dropping like flies—they have declined 60 percent in the last forty years.[2] We see the same massive decline with testosterone levels. As a result, one in five couples has trouble getting pregnant or sustaining a pregnancy. It's pretty dismal, and it's getting worse. *But why?*

In a nutshell, it's because our genes are mismatched to our current environment (so-called evolutionary mismatch). We are maladapted to thrive and procreate in our current environment.

Our environment has changed *more in the last fifty years than it has in the last several thousand years.* New environment = new problems.

The rate of change in our environment has been exponential, and we are running a huge population-wide experiment as a result. The problems we are facing today are brand-new; our parents, grandparents, and great-grandparents didn't face the same chronic disease burden or the same toxic burden or the same infertility burden. It's not just that the solutions are immature; the problem itself is new.

Our environment has drastically changed, and it is causing widespread reverberations. Hormonal and fertility challenges are some of the most profound consequences. Let's dive into each of these environmental shifts in a bit more detail to understand the specific effects on fertility.

TOP FERTILITY BLOCKERS

Poor Nutrition

The way we eat has changed more in the last fifty years than in the previous ten thousand years.[3] We are eating less food and more food-like substances. Processed foods are specifically manufactured to hit our "bliss point," the optimal taste profile that overrides our satiety mechanisms and encourages us to keep coming back for more. Grocery stores are stocked with these hyper-palatable, calorie-dense, and highly processed foods. In most places in the US, food is immediately and abundantly available—morning, noon, and night. Our environment is replete with obesogens, a class of chemicals that predisposes us to weight gain.

Proper nutrition is intimately connected with fertility. Your body will always prioritize survival over procreation; it downregulates reproductive function when it believes there isn't a stable environment to bring a baby into. If you aren't getting proper nutrition, your body perceives this as "famine" and diverts resources away from reproduction.

Like its impact on many other areas of your health, eating a poor, imbalanced diet can impair your fertility. A poor diet can affect your blood sugar levels, your nutrient levels, and your inflammation levels, just to name a few. All of these can interfere with egg and sperm quality. Not surprisingly, women who followed the principles of a fertility diet alongside other healthy lifestyle behaviors decreased ovulatory infertility by 70 percent, and healthier diets have been shown to improve sperm parameters (e.g., sperm count, sperm concentration, and sperm motility) in men with poor semen quality.[4]

In Chapter 12, we will explore the specifics of a fertility-friendly diet. Until then, suffice it to say that balanced nutrition is a critical part of getting pregnant and sustaining a healthy pregnancy.

Environmental Chemicals

Did you know that wildlife researchers have discovered feminized male fish in lakes and rivers around the world? Female egg cells have been found growing inside the testes of smallmouth and largemouth bass.[5] This condition (called intersex) is suspected to be an indicator of exposure to environmental estrogen. These environmental estrogens can come from both natural and synthetic chemicals (such as from pharmaceuticals, pesticides, and personal care products) and can mimic or block sex hormones. In severe cases, intersex conditions can make fish sterile. We are also seeing similar intersex conditions in a variety of other aquatic animals, such as frogs.[6]

These aquatic animals are a harbinger of what's to come. Our waterways are polluted, which means that our environment is polluted. There are eighty-six thousand chemicals monitored by the Environmental Protection Agency's Toxic Substances Control Act Inventory, which is a list of each chemical substance manufactured or processed in the United States, including imports. When the inventory was started in 1975, it contained sixty-two thousand substances, meaning twenty-four thousand chemicals have been introduced to our environment in the last fifty years.[7] We are inundated with more chemicals than our body knows what to do with. It's only a matter of time before this pollution starts affecting humans, and we are already seeing signs that these impacts have started occurring.

In addition to the drop in sperm counts mentioned above, precocious puberty (onset of puberty before age nine) is on the rise in children; we are also seeing an uptick in intersex children exposed to endocrine-disrupting chemicals at key fetal developmental points.[8] This obviously has a profound effect on fertility, but it also has far-reaching consequences for other disease states like cancer.

See Chapter 9 for more on how this toxic load impacts fertility and what you can do about it.

Constant Stress

Stress has increased 20 percent on average in the last thirty years—and that's likely understated.[9] We are more stretched and stressed than ever before. This is relevant for fertility because your sex hormones and your stress hormones are in the same biochemical pathway.

Again, from an evolutionary perspective, your body will always prioritize survival over procreation. Practically speaking, this means that when we are constantly stressed (whether from a long commute or regimented marathon training or significant financial obligations), our bodies divert the raw materials needed to make our sex hormones (e.g., progesterone, testosterone, estrogen) to make our stress hormones (e.g., cortisol, adrenaline) instead. Over time, that means that we don't have the necessary sex hormones to get pregnant or sustain a pregnancy.

Further, stress in early pregnancy has been found to result in localized inflammation in the uterus, reduced production of progesterone (which is essential to maintaining early pregnancy), and increased production of adrenaline (which can directly interfere with development of the embryo). This is all to say that high levels of chronic stress can impact your ability to get pregnant, stay pregnant, and have a healthy pregnancy.

This is also true for males. Elevated, chronic stress levels can impact semen volume and semen quality.[10] In one study, the number of "healthy" sperm was significantly reduced in stressed men compared to reference values. Get this, though: that same study found that the number of "healthy" sperm was significantly higher after stress therapy, indicating a recovery of sperm quality.[11] Luckily, this means that you can manage your stress levels and get your sperm moving and shaking again.

See Chapter 15 for how to combat elevated stress levels.

Sedentary Lifestyle

We are significantly more sedentary than previous generations. We are working more and moving less. According to the American Heart Association:

> People are less active due to technology and better mass transportation. Sedentary jobs have increased 83 percent since 1950; Physically active jobs now make up only about 25 percent of our workforce. That is 50 percent less than 1950. Our average work week is longer. Americans work forty-seven hours a week—164 more hours a year than twenty years ago.[12]

We also have planes, trains, and automobiles, so we don't have to walk more than ten feet on our own if we don't want to. As a result, the majority of adults spend six to eight hours sitting daily, and 45 percent of individuals report no leisure-time activity at all.[13]

For males in particular, certain physical risk factors are associated with sperm anomalies, such as mechanical vibrations, excess heat, and extended sitting periods.[14] Mechanical vibrations can originate from machinery or motorcycles. Excess heat can originate from saunas, steam rooms, or hot tubs, for example. And extended sitting periods often come from desk jobs.

Fortunately, there is something that we can do about it. A recent study showed that exercise improved semen quality and reproductive hormone levels in sedentary obese adults.[15] There are probably several reasons this is the case, including increased cardiovascular capacity, increased antioxidant capacity, and improved blood sugar profiles.[16]

We Are Not Operating under Peak Conditions

Our bodies were designed to procreate in peak conditions; today's environment is a far cry from those peak conditions.

When our body is deficient in key nutrients, especially nutrients needed to sustain a pregnancy, *it downregulates reproductive function*. When our body is constantly stressed (especially if it thinks our environment is unsafe), *it downregulates reproductive function*. When our body is overloaded with toxins (especially if these toxins could poison a growing baby), *it downregulates reproductive function*.

Your body will always prioritize survival over procreation; it downregulates reproductive function when it believes there isn't a safe or stable environment to bring a baby into. And our modern environment triggers these failsafes constantly.

What does that mean practically? That it's harder to get pregnant!

Our reproductive function is the canary in the coal mine. It is exquisitely sensitive to imbalance and adverse conditions. When reproductive function shuts down, it indicates that something is wrong—and will only get worse if we don't address it.

Reproduction is an incredibly robust but delicate process. If our bodies perceive that our environment is unsafe (e.g., due to war) or unstable (e.g., due to famine), our reproductive function will shut off. Though it may seem disconcerting, this "off switch" is a brilliant adaptation. You wouldn't want to bring a baby into a world littered with war and famine, would you? And if you did, that baby would be unlikely to survive. So your body shuts off your ability to conceive and bides its time until conditions improve.

In our modern-day world, though, your body may experience the "unsafe" signal when navigating morning traffic or the "unstable" signal when you try your tenth diet of the month. If anything is off in your body, your reproductive function will feel it first and act accordingly. This may manifest as severe PMS symptoms, adult acne, and even irregular or absent ovulation—all signs of hormonal imbalance, which is a precursor to infertility.

It's time to heed the warning.

Our modern lifestyle is full of fertility blockers. That is abundantly clear. However, we may only be scratching the surface with all the potential implications on our reproductive function. There is also a lot that we still don't understand or haven't fully unpacked. For example, there are suggestions that male sperm-production capability and female ovarian reserve may be influenced while in utero. This is definitely an area ripe for exploration.[17] However, based on the above factors, there are many things that you can do to minimize the effects of these fertility blockers and positively influence both egg and sperm health.

GOING BACK TO BASICS

It's time to go back to basics. In this case, going "back to basics" means understanding the path that's worked for hundreds of thousands of years of human evolution. It means gaining inspiration from the way our ancestors lived and loved (read: procreated). Our ancestors did not experience the same fertility challenges that we are seeing today; they were fertile little buggers. *How can we combine ancient wisdom with modern science to optimize our fertility and the health of future generations?* Lucky for you, that's exactly what I've spent the past several years researching and synthesizing.

In regard to our ancestors, we can ask ourselves, *How did they eat? Move? Connect? Sleep? Play? Relax? What was their pace of life? How did they "do" life?*

By looking at their lives through this lens, we can gain insight into how our bodies are *designed* to operate. What we figure out is that our bodies were carefully and expertly designed to:

- Eat a balanced and varied diet.
- Move regularly.

- Connect deeply with others.
- Sleep fully and soundly.
- Relax on the regular.
- Incorporate play and recreation.

When we consistently experience these things, it signals to our body that we are in a safe, abundant, and welcoming environment. That translates happy messages to our hormones. Safe, abundant, and welcoming environment = green light to procreate.

On the other hand, if our environment feels unsafe, resource-constrained, or hostile, that will convey a yellow or red light to our body with regard to procreation. We can't bring a new life into this world without the nourishment and security to support it.

That being said, our bodies are incredibly resilient. Once you identify what's making you unwell (whether it be toxic food, home care products, relationships), your body can repair itself. It may take time and some detective work, but it's absolutely possible. Your body is designed to procreate— you just need to convince your body that it's safe to do so.

We spend most of our lives trying not to get pregnant. It takes conscious effort and action to completely reorient our lives to trying to get pregnant. It's not always a seamless transition when we decide to turn the faucet back on, so to speak. It takes intention and time, all of which will be discussed in upcoming chapters. We are going to discuss all the ways to align your lifestyle and environment to the ones that your genes were designed for. In Chapter 6, we are going to explore the potential areas that could be out of balance that I've discovered from my years of experience, and I am going to give you a roadmap to get them tested so you know what you're working with.

WHY AM I JUST HEARING ABOUT THIS NOW?

Whenever I talk to individuals about the steps they can be taking to optimally prepare their body, mind, and environment to get and stay pregnant, they always ask the same question: *Why hasn't my doctor told me about this? At this point, you may be wondering the same thing.*

I have two hypotheses to propose:

1. Doctors Don't Have These Tools in Their Toolkit

In general, the majority of doctors have been armed with two main interventional therapies in their arsenal: medication and surgery. In medical school, they were trained to use these two tools very well. However, as the saying goes, if all you have is a hammer, everything looks like a nail. For all medical problems, doctors try to use these same two tools. In the case of chronic disease specifically, we know that these tools are woefully inadequate. Chronic disease is largely a lifestyle problem, not a medical problem; as a result, the solutions need to be lifestyle-related (e.g., diet, exercise, stress management) rather than medical.

The same is true of fertility. Many times, infertility is secondary to chronic disease (whether you know you have a chronic disease or not). Or it is secondary to lifestyle habits or environmental influences that are inconsistent with pregnancy (e.g., high stress, high toxin load). The tools to "treat" fertility may very well be foundational things like diet, stress management, and detoxification, which doctors are not well equipped to address. Such lifestyle interventions are the sweet spot of functionally trained health practitioners—both physicians who have pursued additional training in this field and other kinds of health providers such as nutritionists and health coaches who have similarly been educated in these strategies.

2. Our Current Healthcare Model Isn't Structured to Support Lifestyle Interventions

Lifestyle change, and therefore behavior change, takes time. In some cases, it can require a lot of coaching and troubleshooting. Quite simply, doctors cannot do that kind of hand-holding. Doctors face enormous pressure to see large volumes of patients to meet the needs of their communities and satisfy the requirements of their institutions. Their priority is to keep us alive and manage disease. Keeping us "well" requires a different kind of medical strategy entirely. Thus, they simply do not have the luxury of time to spend on the in-depth discussions that are required to counsel each patient through making lifestyle changes. The structure is not set up to allow them to do so. That's partly why the whole health coaching industry has sprung up to fill this gap.

All of this being said, we can't be too hard on our doctors. Most of them are well-intentioned clinicians trying to do their best for their patients with the tools that they have available to them and in a system that's increasingly complex to navigate. (See Chapter 8 to learn more about how to work with your doctor at a preconception visit.) However, I want you to know that there is another way, and I want to show you the path to get there.

CHAPTER SUMMARY

- Just as our environment is obesogenic (predisposes us to obesity), it is also infertile-genic (predisposes us to infertility). Our genes were designed for conception, but our modern environment was not. It requires corrective action to offset this.

- Our environment has changed more in the last fifty years than it has in the last ten thousand years, and this is causing widespread reverberations, particularly on fertility. Impaired reproductive health is the canary in the coal mine.

- Top fertility blockers include poor nutrition, environmental chemicals, constant stress, and sedentary lifestyles.

- Your body will always prioritize survival over procreation. We need to go back to basics to align ourselves to the conditions for reproductive success: a safe, stable, and resource-abundant environment.

THE SOLUTION

The Case for
Pre-Pregnancy Preparation

*"Having a baby is like building a house—you have
to prepare a good, strong foundation before you
start the actual construction. The foundation
from which a baby grows is a woman's egg, or
ovum, and a man's sperm. To give a baby the
best start in life both partners have to be as
healthy as possible before they try to conceive."*
—The Pre-Pregnancy Planner

Experts agree that the optimal time for couples to
improve their health is *before* becoming pregnant. In
fact, the choices you and your reproductive partner
make before pregnancy can be even more impactful
than the ones you make during pregnancy. By taking

action on potential health issues and risks before pregnancy, you can prevent problems that might affect you or your baby later. The healthier you are when you conceive, the better foundation you set for your child's future health.

The Preconception Period: The Forgotten Developmental Stage

We treat conception as a single moment in time. Today, preconception healthcare is invisible. Reproductive care for women is either focused on contraception (preventing a pregnancy) or prenatal care (managing a pregnancy); there is nothing in between. This approach is insufficient, and it's causing harm to our mothers, our babies, our families. We are missing the entire intervening period after contraception ends and when conception begins. It's most effective when we treat this as its own unique period of time—*the preconception period*. A *pre-mester*, if you will!

Ideally, preconception begins the moment a couple decides they want to have kids. Practically speaking, it involves the approximately one-year period prior to conception. According to the CDC:

> If you are trying to have a baby or are just thinking about it, it is not too early to start getting ready for pregnancy. Preconception health and health care focus on things you can do before and between pregnancies to increase the chances of having a healthy baby...whether this is your first, second, or sixth baby.[1]

As I shared in the Introduction, planning and preparing for pregnancy *before* you want to get pregnant makes it easier to get pregnant and increases the likelihood of having a healthy baby.

The natural next question is: why? In the next two chapters, we will explore the answers to this question.

(4)

START PREPARING EARLIER

Parenting Begins before Conception

THE DELICATE DANCE OF CONCEPTION

Conception is a miraculous thing, but it is also very tenuous. A lot of successive things need to go right in order to make a baby. In natural conception (without the aid of ART), here's how it plays out:

For Females

- You need to be *ovulating regularly*, which means your ovaries release an egg each month.
- That egg needs to make its way from the ovary into the fallopian tube without any obstructions.
- Then that egg needs to have the sustenance and wherewithal to wait for "the one" (i.e., the triumphant sperm that reaches and penetrates the egg first).

For Males

- You need to have *enough sperm* (a high enough sperm count) to give you a fighting chance of making a baby.
- Enough of those *sperm need to be in good shape* (morphology) to tip the odds in your favor.
- Those *sperm need to be vibrant enough* (motility) to make the long, hard journey from your partner's vagina to her cervix and eventually to her fallopian tubes.
- Finally, one superhero sperm needs to find the egg and *penetrate it* within around twenty-four hours of ovulation (fertilization).

For the Fertilized Egg

- The fertilized egg (zygote) needs to make its way *from the fallopian tube into the uterus* without any obstructions.
- The zygote needs to *divide in an orderly and appropriate fashion.*
- The zygote needs to *implant itself in the uterine lining,* which must be thick and cozy enough to support it.
- Then the embryo needs to *grow without obstruction* to term.

As you can see, there are many stops on the train that can go wrong. Suboptimal health for either partner increases the probability of derailing the train. That's why it's incredibly important to prepare in advance to provide as smooth and seamless of a path for the train to follow as possible.

WHY DOES PREPARING FOR PREGNANCY MAKE IT EASIER TO GET PREGNANT?

We need adequate time to *undo* the effects of the fertility blockers in our modern environment to essentially coax our bodies back into the natural state that's receptive to conception.

Most people are living lives that are incompatible with optimal fertility. As we discussed in the last section, our grandmothers and great-grandmothers didn't struggle with the same epidemic of infertility that our peers are struggling with. More sleep, less stress, lower toxic burden, higher-quality nutrition—these sound like anomalies to us today, but they were the foundation of how generations before us lived and thrived. Ample time is needed to remove toxin exposures and amplify the body's detoxification pathways, boost nutritional stores, and establish hormone balance prior to conception. Getting all of this in order in advance makes it easier to get pregnant when you are ready.

PRECONCEPTION PLANNING: NOT JUST FOR YOUR FIRST RODEO

Preparing to get pregnant is not only relevant for a first-time pregnancy. This preparation process applies to *each pregnancy*. In fact, you may be more likely to need extra preparation time after a previous pregnancy. The two things I see most commonly after a previous pregnancy are:

- Imbalanced hormones: Hormones are more likely to be imbalanced after the roller coaster that is pregnancy, postpartum, and breastfeeding (if applicable).
- Nutrient depletion: Nutrients are more likely to be depleted after growing and nurturing another human.

Pre-pregnancy wellness testing (which we will discuss in the next section) can help you understand whether your hormones have settled back into a balanced state or whether they may need a little extra attention. It can also tell you your nutrient status so you'll know if you need to focus on replenishing your body through nourishing foods and targeted supplements.

HOW MUCH TIME WILL I NEED?

The time required to prepare will depend on your baseline health, which we will discuss more in the next section. For most couples, I recommend at least three to twelve months before trying to conceive. Of course, if you have underlying health problems or haven't been living a particularly healthy lifestyle, it may take longer than this to upgrade your health, but three to twelve months is the minimum time I recommend to prepare. If you're eager, you can give yourself even more time; technically, it's never too early to get ready for a healthy pregnancy and baby.

Here are five top reasons you need ample time to prepare.

1. For Egg and Sperm Development

Women are born with a store of eggs at birth. These eggs mature somewhat in utero but then exist in a state of "suspended animation" or a "Sleeping Beauty–like state" for much of your life. Each month, a subset of these eggs is selected for maturation, and they exit this "Sleeping Beauty" state to finish their final maturation process. It takes around twelve months to fully mature an egg to be ovulated. It is really only during this period of maturation, when eggs "awaken" from a Sleeping Beauty state that they are most susceptible to the environmental conditions around them. The last stage of egg maturation (the three- to four-month window prior to ovulation) is when egg quality is most impacted. That is why this three- to twelve-month time frame prior to ovulation is particularly important when it comes to the health of your maturing eggs and, therefore, your baby. It's not that your lifestyle prior to that doesn't matter at all (it does), but it's really this one-year period (and in particular, those last three to four months prior to ovulation) that's most impactful when it comes to egg health.

In addition, it takes about three months (around seventy-four days) for new sperm to fully develop. Males are constantly making new sperm, and there is ample opportunity to improve their vibrancy as a result.

Your lifestyle during the three to twelve months prior to conception sets the stage for your egg or sperm health, which will literally make up the building blocks of your baby's cells. Depending on your starting point, it may take several egg or sperm development cycles to upgrade egg and sperm quality and improve outcomes.

2. For Nutrient Stores

Depending on your starting point, it can take a while to upgrade your eating habits and build up your nutrient stores. You want to give yourself plenty of runway to implement these changes and for your body to reflect them.

If you were on hormonal birth control or other medications prior to conceiving, these may have depleted some of your nutrient stores. If you have recently experienced prolonged, heightened stress, that may have depleted some of your nutrient stores. If you have ongoing gastrointestinal issues such as gas, bloating, or constipation that may signal you are not digesting and assimilating your food properly, this could mean that some of your nutrient stores are inadequate.

These are just a few examples of cases where you may have depleted stores of nutrients that are necessary for fetal development. For females, that lack of nutrients may have manifested as fatigue, lethargy, mood challenges, or even lowered immune function, but when you introduce a baby into that equation, your nutrient needs increase drastically, and low nutrient stores are taxed even further. Your nutrient stores have to provide for *both* you and your growing baby. It can take several months to build up these nutrient stores, so it's imperative to start as early as possible to figure out your nutritional status and address any potential gaps. We will get into many more juicy details about nutrition in Chapter 12, so stay tuned.

3. For Detoxification

We have a whole chapter dedicated to this topic, so I won't go into detail here. Suffice it to say, it can take quite some time to identify sources of toxic exposure in air, water, food, personal care products, and home care products and swap them for less-toxic alternatives—and then for your body to reflect those upgrades.

4. For Management of Chronic Health Conditions

If you have chronic health conditions such as diabetes, thyroid disease, or anxiety, it is imperative to make sure that these are well controlled before conception. This process may also include discussing medication or dosage changes with your doctor to ensure that they are fertility and pregnancy safe. This discussion of managing your health conditions will be a central part of your preconception visit (see Chapter 8 for more details).

5. For Cycle Tracking (Females)

Once you've gone off hormonal birth control, it's time to get to know your monthly cycle. When does it start? How long does it last? What types of symptoms do you experience, if any?

As a reminder from Chapter 2, birth control essentially cuts off communication between your brain and your ovaries. It can take some time for this communication mechanism to kick back in and, therefore, for your period and ovulation to normalize. We will discuss this more in Chapter 11, but restoring a normal period after hormonal birth control is a critical part of conception preparation and can take up to a year.

For all these reasons, preparing in advance is the way to go for optimal outcomes—for both you and your future baby.[1]

DO I WANT KIDS?

This may seem like an odd question in a book about preparing to get pregnant, but as with all things preconception, I believe in the importance of being intentional.

Preconception begins the moment you decide that you want to have kids. But have you really decided? Childbearing in today's society is not a family or economic obligation but a personal choice. Having children or not having children are both viable options. However, making a considered decision means being able to evaluate both possibilities fully and objectively.

There are two main questions to consider:

1. Do I want to have kids?
   a. What are my motivations for having a child?
   b. What are my expectations of myself and my partner? Are these expectations reasonable?
   c. What will change once I become a parent (e.g., in my career, in my relationship, in my identity)? What will stay the same?
   d. What do I think being a parent will be like? Who do I envision myself being as a parent?
   e. What do I think my child(ren) will be like?

f. Do I feel pressure to have kids from someone or something else (e.g., parents, friends, religion)?

g. What would my future look like without children?

2. When do I want to have kids?
   a. Am I physically ready for kids?
   b. Am I emotionally ready for kids (e.g., have I dealt with past trauma or challenging relationships with my own parents)?
   c. Am I financially ready for kids?
   d. Are my partner and I on the same page about timing?
   e. Is my physical space compatible with having children right now?
   f. Is my job/career compatible with having children right now?
   g. Are there any things I want to do or milestones I want to reach before having children?

After talking with hundreds of couples trying to conceive, I've found that most would prefer to spend more time preparing to conceive than trying to conceive. There's just something more inherently pressure-inducing once you start "trying." How about you? Would you rather spend more time preparing to conceive or trying to conceive? If you said preparing, then have I got a checklist for you! I am going to walk you through that step-by-step in the next section. But before we get there, an important exploration of legacy in the next chapter...

CHAPTER SUMMARY

- Conception is a miraculous but tenuous process. A lot of successive things need to go right to make a baby.

- Healthier parents conceive more easily. Pre-pregnancy preparation can increase the chances of getting pregnant.

- The nine months of pregnancy is not enough prep time for optimal health outcomes—for mom, for baby, for family. It can take up to a year to properly prepare for pregnancy, depending on your starting point. This includes optimizing egg and sperm development, repleting nutrient stores, reducing toxic exposures, managing chronic conditions, and restoring a normal menstrual cycle.

- Optimal pre-pregnancy preparation involves both reproductive partners in the process.

- Pre-pregnancy preparation is as relevant for a first-time pregnancy as it is for a fifth.

(5)

BUILD GENERATIONAL HEALTH

The Legacy You Leave Your Children

n the last chapter, we discussed how preparing for pregnancy increases the chances of getting pregnant. In this chapter, we are going to answer an even more profound question: *why does preparing for pregnancy increase the likelihood of having a healthy baby?*

THE LINK BETWEEN PRECONCEPTION HEALTH AND PRENATAL AND POSTNATAL HEALTH

This may seem reductive, but if we don't know what we are aiming at, it's hard to get there. Let's start with some definitions. In traditional terms, health is the absence of disease. Wellness is more than the mere absence of disease; it's an optimal, vibrant state of being. I think we can do better than health, but let's at least start there!

At minimum, a healthy pregnancy is full term and free from complications for mom, like gestational diabetes, pregnancy-induced hypertension, or preeclampsia. At minimum, a healthy baby is full term and normal birthweight and does not suffer from birth defects, developmental disabilities/delays, or other health conditions.

Of course, mom's health and baby's health are closely related. Let's take an example. Nutritional stores in preconception can affect growth in pregnancy. If a mother enters pregnancy deficient in key nutrients (e.g., vitamin D, zinc, iron), the baby's growth is likely to be suboptimal, resulting in intrauterine growth restriction (IGR). Intrauterine growth restriction can also occur as a result of a variety of maternal health conditions, including hypertension, diabetes, chronic kidney disease, heart disease, and infection. It can also be secondary to smoking, alcohol, and drug use. With IGR, the baby doesn't get the nutrients and oxygen needed to grow and develop organs and tissues properly. As a result, the baby may be born small for gestational age (SGA). Infants born SGA due to fetal growth restriction are at increased risk of short-term complications such as infection, hypothermia (difficulty regulating body temperature), low or high blood sugar levels, hypocalcemia (low calcium levels), polycythemia (too many red blood cells), and sepsis, as well as long-term complications such as learning difficulties, hypertension, stroke, heart disease, and dementia.[1]

In another example, gestational diabetes increases the likelihood of delivering babies large for gestational age (born too large). Large babies also increase the likelihood of C-section deliveries, which come with their own set of potential complications. Babies born large for gestational age (LGA) carry an increased risk for adult expression of obesity, diabetes, hypertension, and cardiovascular disease.[2] Here's the punch line: complications in pregnancy have a *high association* with chronic disease across the lifespan of that child. There is a clear link between health in the prenatal period (before birth) and the postnatal period (after birth).

What we are now starting to realize is that there is an *even earlier link* between the preconception period and the prenatal and postnatal periods. The preconception period affects the prenatal period. The prenatal period affects the postnatal period. There are profound knock-on effects from one period to the next. All of these effects are connected and compound over time. We have been missing one of the most foundational developmental periods by completely skipping over preconception. We've known for a while that the first one thousand days of life is a critical developmental period for babies, and science is now demonstrating that that critical developmental window extends even prior to conception.

Studies show that exposures and interventions such as diet, exercise, and other lifestyle behaviors can have long-lasting consequences not only for pregnancy outcomes but also for long-term health across generations.[3] The good news is that many of the factors that increase the likelihood of a baby being born preterm, small for gestational age, or large for gestational age are modifiable. These modifiable lifestyle factors are addressable by you and your reproductive partner even before you conceive.

To explain these linkages further, let's do a brief tour of genetics and epigenetics.

GENETICS AND EPIGENETICS

As recently as a few decades ago, the study of genetics was a brand-new field, and scientists believed that your genes were your destiny. Genetic predeterminism was the predominant theory of health for generations. Predeterminism is the idea that all events, including human actions, are decided in advance (or *predetermined*). In the context of healthcare, it means that the development of individual health is predetermined by heredity. In the nature versus nurture debate, it puts all of the eggs in the "nature" category—you are born with a certain set of genes, and those genes determine your destiny—and *there ain't nothin' you can do about it.*

For some of us, that message may have been comforting. *If my fate is sealed, I might as well have this double fudge sundae...or these delectable fried chicken wings...or this divine Bordeaux. After all, it doesn't really matter.* For others, that message may have been incredibly disempowering. *What's the point of eating well and exercising consistently if it doesn't ultimately make a difference?*

With the advent of new scientific and technological breakthroughs, however, we now know that the "genetics is king" theory is simply not true. Recent studies have shown that our epigenome is influenced by our habitat and lifestyle. Cutting-edge research suggests that it's not just genes themselves that are relevant, but rather *the environment the genes exist in* that dictates what happens to the genes.[4]

In fact, Eric Lander, PhD, geneticist and one of the leaders of the Human Genome Project, so eloquently said:

> The greatest danger is a mistaken sense of genetic determinism—that people will think that because genes play a role in something, they determine everything. We see, again and again, people saying, "It's all genetic. I can't do anything about it." That's nonsense. To say that something has a genetic component does not mean it's unchangeable. Environmental factors play a huge role.[5]

There you have it—from someone who spent a huge part of his career advancing genetic science. Genes absolutely play a fundamental role in health, but they are not the whole story; frankly, they're not even most of the story.

Let's take a step back for a moment to distinguish between genetics and epigenetics a bit more.

The genome is the sum total of all of the genes in your body. Our genes determine our characteristics (e.g., hair color, eye color, height). Unfortunately, it's not as simple as a one-to-one cause-and-effect: one gene can affect several traits, and one trait may be affected by several genes. However, for our purposes, it's just important to understand that our genes are determined at birth, our genes are fixed, and our genes influence our characteristics.

The epigenome, on the other hand, is a multitude of chemical compounds that can tell the genome what to do.[6] If the genome is the light bulb, the epigenome is the light switch that turns the light on or off. Or if you find this analogy more helpful, if the genome is the hardware, the epigenome is the software. Therefore, the epigenome is actually what affects the expression of genes. Most importantly, the epigenome is not fixed (like the genome) and can change throughout a person's lifetime. Changes to the epigenome can be positive (e.g., as a result of exercise or meditation) or negative (e.g., as a result of smoking or a poor diet). Our environment shapes how our genes (genetics) are expressed (epigenetics).

A person's environment, including their diet, lifestyle, and exposure to certain nutrients, chemicals, and stressors, can influence the expression of certain genes, which can then alter their risk of developing certain health conditions down the road. Your genes and your environment can interact in ways that can change how your genes are expressed (e.g., switching particular genes on or off, dialing gene expression up or down) without altering the underlying sequence of DNA. These "on-off" switches, for example, determine which proteins are expressed in the body; the expressed proteins then manifest as either health or disease. As a result, your health is not just about your genetic blueprint but rather the interplay of your genetic blueprint *and* your environmental influences.

In case this helps put a finer point on things, genetics and epigenetics can best be explained in the context of twins. Identical twins always have the same genes, but they often will have different epigenetics (the expression of their genes).

Why does this matter?

These scientific findings have ushered in the era of self-determinism, which means that you have control over your health decisions and therefore your health outcomes. How much control? The latest research estimates that 25 percent of the variance in health and longevity comes from genetics, and the remaining 75 percent comes from environmental factors (including things like diet, exercise, stress, and exposure to toxins).[7] An overwhelming majority of our health is influenced by our environment (read: our physical surroundings as well as our lifestyle choices), not our inherited genetic makeup. In other words, the vast majority of your health outcomes are in your control.

INHERITED EPIGENETICS

Importantly for parents-to-be, these epigenetic influences start in the womb, the very first "environment" your child ever experiences. What's even more wild is that if certain parts of your genetic blueprint are turned on or off by a certain environmental factor (say smoking, for instance) then the impact that this environmental factor has on your genes can also be passed down to your children and your children's children. We now know that your epigenome (the environmental influence on your genetic blueprint) is inheritable from generation to generation, just like your genome (the genetic blueprint itself).

Shanna Swan says it well in *Count Down*:

> The food we eat, the air we breathe, the products we use, and the emotions we feel have the potential to influence not only how our own genes are expressed but also how those of our unborn descendants might behave in the

future…our lifestyles and environments can have ripple effects on the health and development of our unborn children and grandchildren through mechanisms that foster cellular memory and can be maintained across several generations.[8]

In other words, the decisions you make today have the ability to impact not only your children but your children's children and potentially even your children's children's children and beyond. Environmental exposures lead to heritable epigenetic changes.

Mark Hyman, MD, founder of The UltraWellness Center and best-selling author, explains this well:

> If your grandmother ate too much sugar, or smoked, or was exposed to mercury from too much sushi, the genetic modifications she incurred from this exposure could affect you. Her epigenome would carry an increased risk of disease that could be passed down from generation to generation.[9]

Similarly, if your grandmother meditated daily, ate foods grown from her garden, walked everywhere and laughed a lot, her epigenome would likely carry a decreased risk of disease that would be passed on to you. *Pretty incredible, isn't it?*

Recent animal and human studies have shown how this epigenetic memory is passed through generations, affecting things as diverse as the risk of high blood sugar, the risk of obesity, cognitive development, susceptibility to stress, and even propensity for binge eating.[10] These epigenetic changes do not affect the actual DNA sequence of genes, but they can change how that DNA is packaged and how those genes are ultimately expressed.

You may be wondering why these epigenetic changes get transferred between generations.

It's adaptation at its best. It takes many, many generations for gene sequences to change, so in order to pass on adaptive behaviors from one generation to the next, the body makes epigenetic changes. Since these epigenetic changes can happen within a single generation, passing these traits on can give children a "pre-adaptive" advantage to changes in the environment. This is precisely why the life experiences and lifestyle of one generation can impact the development of subsequent generations.

You may be wondering how exactly these epigenetics are passed to children. *Wait for it…wait for it…it's through egg and sperm!* Egg and sperm contain DNA with both genetic and epigenetic material. Egg and sperm are essentially microcosms of your whole health—a "mini me." At the point of conception, the egg and sperm come together and combine their DNA to make their baby's DNA. This DNA contains both the hardware (genetics) and software (epigenetics) of your baby's future operating system (i.e., health). This is where generational health comes in—and your ability to influence it.

There are tons of studies that are coming out now to demonstrate what does and does not affect our epigenetics; this is a constantly evolving area of science, so stay tuned. Suffice it to say, there is still a lot we don't know, but we do know this: you are largely in control of your gene expression! What you eat, how you move, how much you sleep, and how you manage stress are all epigenetic modulators, and they are all under your control.

Don't go getting all panicky on me. I know this can feel like a lot of pressure. Your decisions may affect not only you but your baby and your baby's baby? That's a lot to take in.

This information is meant to be empowering, not overwhelming. You have the power to change your health for the better, and the good decisions that you make today and every day also set the stage for the amazing children that you will have one day.

Here are the two big takeaways: first, whatever genetic predisposition your parents gave you, you have the power to modulate it through epigenetics. Second, you have a lot of power to transmute goodness to your kids. As mentioned earlier, epigenetic markers in egg and sperm set the stage for your baby's health later in life. A part of your child's future health is genetically influenced, while many other parts are informed by the condition of your body and your reproductive partner's body before conception. *Your health status when you conceive sets the stage for your child's health. The healthier you are when you conceive, the better foundation you set for your child's lifelong health.*

Taking a step back from the nitty-gritty science for a moment, what this means is that your health (and by extension, the health of your children) is not set in stone; you can take actions, starting today, to improve your health and the health of your family for generations to come.

ARE YOU IN THE STATE OF HEALTH THAT YOU'D WANT TO PASS ON TO A CHILD?

People choose to have children for many reasons—to embody love for one another, to participate in one of life's great adventures, to infuse life with more meaning. One of the most powerful and far-reaching reasons for having children is also legacy.

Legacy is something handed down from one generation to the next. For many people, it's a way for them to "live on" through their offspring.

What type of legacy do you want to leave your children?

Most parents would say that they want to leave their children better off than they were. They wouldn't want their children to make the same mistakes that they did—in life, in love, in education, in business. They would want their children to pick up where they left off and get even more out of life.

Many people think of legacy as financial in nature. But there are so many more components to legacy—it's the values you teach your children, the love you communicate to them, the biases you consciously or unconsciously share with them, the beliefs that drive you that they internalize, the fears that shape you that also shape them, and the hopes and dreams that you pursue that influence their worldview.

I'd like to offer an even more expanded view of legacy.

Legacy is also the health you leave your children. This is called generational health.

What you do today has the power to impact not only your children's health, but also your children's children's health. Talk about legacy.

Health is one of the best gifts that you can endow your children with, and it lasts a lifetime. Why not give your child the gift of incredible health starting today? Healthy people are happier, more productive, more social, and more able to embrace life. Health is a gift that keeps on giving. *What better gift can a parent bestow on a child than the foundation of vibrant health?*

DO IT FOR THE KIDS...
BUT NOT JUST FOR THE KIDS

This entire book is about preconception—becoming a better you so that you can set the stage for a healthier family. Now I'm going to tell you to be selfish for a moment. Why? Because fertility is a marker of future health. As Shanna Swan writes in *Count Down*:

> Low sperm count, recurrent miscarriages, and reproductive disorders, such as endometriosis and polycystic ovary syndrome (PCOS), can have profound repercussions for a man's or woman's long-term health and even lead to premature mortality.[11]

Studies are showing that "infertility may be a harbinger for future health risk in women, including early mortality. Fertility status itself could serve as an early biomarker...for risk stratification later in life."[12] Ovaries and testes are not just reproductive organs—they are also endocrine organs, which means they have far-reaching effects on overall health. Men with infertility also have an earlier mortality than their more fertile peers.

In *Count Down*, Shanna Swan highlights several of the health risks correlated with infertility for both men and women, including:

- Women diagnosed with infertility are at higher risk for hormone-sensitive cancers. Those who underwent fertility testing and treatment also have an approximately 20 percent increased risk of developing other types of cancer— uterine, ovarian, thyroid, liver, and pancreatic cancers, as well as leukemia.

- Polycystic ovary syndrome (PCOS) is often correlated with insulin resistance and metabolic syndrome, which in turn increases the risk for cardiovascular disease.

- Males with low sperm concentrations have a 30 percent higher risk of developing diabetes and a 48 percent higher risk of developing ischemic heart disease. Low sperm concentration is also associated with increased cancer risk.

- Males with lower testosterone levels not only struggle with fertility but also show increased risk for cardiovascular disease, as well as "muscle loss, increased abdominal fat, weakened bones, erectile dysfunction, and memory, mood, and energy problems."[13]

Reproductive health is the canary in the coal mine. It is an extension of overall health. You can use this time period as an excuse to prioritize yourself. Because it's not just about being a healthy

> parent—it's also about being a healthy person.
> And a thriving coworker, community member, boss,
> employee, friend, sister, and/or brother.

CHAPTER SUMMARY

- The preconception period affects the prenatal period. The prenatal period affects the postnatal period. It's all connected. Complications in pregnancy have a high association with chronic disease across the lifespan.

- The vast majority of health outcomes are driven by epigenetics, not genetics. Epigenetics are modifiable, largely through diet, supplementation, and lifestyle interventions.

- Healthier parents give birth to healthier babies. Optimizing pre-pregnancy wellness increases the chances of having a healthy baby.

- You have the power to give your future children the gift of generational health. Your epigenome (the environmental influence on your genetic blueprint) is inheritable from generation to generation, just like your genome (the genetic blueprint itself). The healthier you are when you conceive, the better foundation you set for your child's lifelong health.

THE PRE-PREGNANCY CHECKLIST

For many couples today, the baby planning process starts and ends with deciding when to stop using birth control. The process usually looks like this:

1. Stop hormonal birth control.
2. Start prenatal vitamins.

As we discussed in earlier chapters, the rising rates of both infertility and reproductive anxiety suggest that this level of planning is insufficient—and it's causing a lot of unnecessary pain and suffering. There is another way. You can give yourself the gift of preparation *before* you actively start trying to conceive.

Would you like to become pregnant in the next year? If so, without further ado, here is the full pre-pregnancy checklist to optimize your chances of a healthy conception, pregnancy, and baby. It does involve stopping hormonal birth control and starting prenatal vitamins, but that's just the beginning.

The checklist is chronological, starting approximately one year prior to trying to conceive (TTC), and is divided into two main sections: Information Gathering and Interventions. In the Information Gathering stage, you will gain an understanding of your baseline health status, which will help you understand what you are currently working with as you contemplate conception and parenthood. In the Interventions stage, you will proactively address the top fertility blockers, as well as take corrective action to address any yellow or red flags that were identified in the Information Gathering stage that could interfere with fertility, a healthy pregnancy, or a healthy baby.

Information Gathering Stage
One year before TTC
- Get your preconception lab testing done (Chapter 6).
- Encourage your reproductive partner to get their preconception lab testing done (Chapter 6).
- Consider whether genetic testing is right for you and your reproductive partner (Chapter 7).
- Schedule a preconception visit with your doctor (Chapter 8).

Intervention Stage
Nine months before TTC

- Minimize potentially harmful environmental exposures that can affect fertility and pregnancy (Chapter 9).
- Rightsize your body composition for conception and pregnancy (Chapter 10).
- For females, discontinue hormonal birth control, if applicable, and switch to an alternate form of contraception. Regulate your menstrual cycle and start tracking ovulation (Chapter 11).

Six months before TTC

- Adopt a fertility-friendly diet (Chapter 12).
- Start taking preconception supplementation (Chapter 13).
- Adopt a fertility-friendly movement plan (Chapter 14).
- Rerun preconception lab tests and follow up with your doctor on any previous findings.

Three months before TTC

- Get your mental game in order (Chapter 15).
- Schedule a dental cleaning if you haven't had one in the last six months (Chapter 8).

TTC

- Start trying (Chapter 16)!

As you can see from the comprehensiveness of this checklist, preconception preparation is not just for people who are unhealthy or have medical problems. It's *for everyone*. It's an opportunity to take a look at your life and health and identify things that could be improved to give you a better chance at a healthy conception, pregnancy, and baby. Proper preconception care is designed to improve the pre-pregnancy wellness of both parents in order to achieve a healthy pregnancy with a healthy child.

> *Please note: This checklist is meant to be a guide. It's comprehensive but not exhaustive. It's also not meant to be prescriptive. It's meant to be a jumping-off point for you and your reproductive partner to get the preconception party started. If you've already started trying to conceive and you are just coming across this checklist now, it's okay. You can start upgrading your lifestyle today. The same applies if you are currently undergoing IVF or IUI—any upgrades that you make can increase your probability of success.*
>
> *For you overachievers out there, yes, you can start earlier. Finding out your pre-pregnancy wellness baseline is a great place to start so you know what you're working with. In my clinical practice, I found that swapping to fertility-friendly products, upgrading diet, and restoring a normal menstrual cycle often took the most time for clients, so if you're looking to get going, those are areas that I would consider prioritizing.*

Ready? Let's dive in.

INFORMATION GATHERING STAGE

How Do I Know If I'm Ready to Conceive?

In some senses, you are never "ready" to become a parent. There are so many things that you can't adequately prepare for until they happen. It's on-the-job-training in its truest form. However, you can still anticipate, plan, and prepare in advance.

If you were training for a marathon, you would probably ask yourself, *Have I trained enough? Am I ready for this race?*

If you were applying to a job, you would probably ask yourself, *Am I qualified enough? Can I handle the demands of this job?*

Similarly, when it comes to pregnancy, we can start asking ourselves, *Am I ready for this? Physically? Emotionally? Financially?* The pre-pregnancy checklist is designed to help guide you through this process. In this section, we are going to focus on how to assess your starting point. In the next section, we will discuss what to do about it. First assess; then act.

Fertility Doesn't Have to Be a Black Box

This first section on assessment consists of two parts:

1. Lab work (pre-pregnancy wellness testing, genetic carrier screening)
2. Preconception visit

Lab work: Your fertility doesn't have to be a black box until you try to conceive and find out that something's off. Your fertility is an extension of your overall health. We can get a sense for the likelihood of a successful conception and pregnancy by looking at a broad set of biomarkers. These biomarkers are all key performance indicators (KPIs) for your fertility, and they can be measured *before* you start trying to conceive. You can figure out your pre-pregnancy wellness baseline so you know what you're working with. This applies to both females and males hoping to conceive.

Preconception visit: We can pair this lab work on your pre-pregnancy wellness baseline with an overall look at your personal and family health history. This deep dive will give you an understanding of potential risk factors—and what you can do about them.

Together, establishing your pre-pregnancy wellness baseline through lab work and determining your risk factors through a preconception visit will set you up well for optimizing your health and the health of your future family.

6

IS YOUR BODY BABY-READY?

Establish Your Pre-Pregnancy Wellness Baseline with Lab Testing

" think I'm healthy. I eat well. I exercise regularly. I feel pretty good overall. *But I sometimes wonder—am I really?*" Julie is a physical therapist, so she has a pretty good baseline understanding of health and wellness, but she was coming to me as she planned to conceive and was starting to wonder whether "good enough" in previous chapters of her life was good enough as she planned to build her family.

This is something I hear often.

Do you ever wonder if there is more you could be doing? You may eat well, exercise regularly, and do your best to limit stress. *But how do you really know if you're doing enough and if what you're doing is working?* Sure, maybe you can rely on how you feel. That's a decent indicator. But is it enough? *How do you know if your body is ready to conceive?*

INTRODUCING THE "BABY-READY BODY"

Every spring, there are tons of articles that go something like this: "6 weeks to your best bikini body," "35 foods to get you bikini ready," or "How to get a bikini-ready body."

I'd like to introduce you to another body type: a "baby-ready body." A baby-ready body is the best possible shape that your body can be in to conceive and carry a healthy pregnancy to term. For a male partner, it is the best possible shape for your body to create optimal sperm for conception. I'm not just talking about your physical shape either, though that does play a critical role. This means getting your body, mind, and environment in tip-top shape for baby-making.

How do you know when you have a "baby-ready body"?

Historically, the only way to know was to get pregnant and have a baby. You only know after you try. But that approach seems outdated.

Instead, let's focus on a new concept called *pre-pregnancy* wellness. Pre-pregnancy wellness is the state of your health prior to getting pregnant (usually one year beforehand) that influences your fertility and the health of your future pregnancy and baby. Understanding your pre-pregnancy wellness helps us to identify any potential issues that may hamper your ability to get pregnant, have a healthy pregnancy, and have a healthy baby.

Your body gives you a lot of information if you know what to look and listen for. However, pre-pregnancy wellness is about more than how you intuitively feel. There are lab tests that can check what is happening at a cellular level.

We can measure a key set of biomarkers that are important for healthy reproduction. This goes beyond just measuring your hormones to measuring your overall health. Think of these biomarkers as KPIs, or key performance indicators. In business, KPIs are metrics that are tracked to determine the trajectory of the business (e.g., sales, new customer sign-ups, retention rate). Your pre-pregnancy wellness status is a KPI for your health and, by extension, your fertility.

Conceiving a healthy baby is one type of KPI for your fertility. However, there are other KPIs for fertility that we can measure *far before* you even try to conceive. Pre-pregnancy wellness testing gives us a much earlier set of indicators of what you are working with.

In this chapter, we are going to cover the specific biomarkers to test to determine your baseline pre-pregnancy wellness. Determining places of imbalance early on will allow you to make the necessary interventions for optimal fertility and pregnancy outcomes.

If you're intrigued but not quite ready to dive into lab testing, I recommend taking Poplin's qualitative baby-readiness assessment as an initial starting point. This assessment will give you a quick read on what factors can impact fertility and pregnancy and where you may need some extra TLC. Go to *quiz.getpoplin.com* to get started.

WHY TEST?

"If you can't measure it, you can't improve it."

—PETER DRUCKER

The importance of testing for establishing your pre-pregnancy baseline has two parts:

1. You don't know *what* needs to change unless you measure it (and thus identify an imbalance).
2. You don't know *how* to change something unless you measure progress against your efforts.

Being proactive about monitoring your health is critical for early intervention. Here's why: if you wait until you experience overt symptoms of disease, it's already too late. In fact, the majority of people with abnormal preconception labs either have no symptoms or think what they are experiencing is normal. This is precisely why it's so important to get screened *in advance* of a potential pregnancy.

Let me explain why this is, according to the CDC's timeline of disease progression.[1] Let's look at a disease process in an individual over time, if left untreated.

The disease process begins after an exposure or an accumulation of disease-causing factors in a susceptible host. Once the disease process is initiated, pathological changes start to occur.

The second stage in the process, called the stage of subclinical disease (or latency period), extends from the time of exposure to the onset of disease symptoms. In this stage, disease is asymptomatic (no symptoms) or inapparent (mild symptoms). For some chronic conditions, this subclinical period can last years.

The transition from subclinical disease to clinical disease is marked by the onset of symptoms. This is when most people head to the doctor and get a diagnosis of disease.

Here's the thing: though disease is not obvious during the subclinical period, certain pathological changes may be detectable with lab testing. Effective screening programs attempt to identify the disease process during the subclinical phase because early intervention is likely to be more effective than treatment after the disease has progressed and become symptomatic. Spoiler alert: this is what pre-pregnancy testing is all about!

In certain individuals, the disease process may never progress to clinically apparent illness; it may fester under the surface for years. According to the CDC, "Because the spectrum of disease can include asymptomatic and mild cases, the cases of illness diagnosed by clinicians in the community often represent only the tip of the iceberg. Many additional cases may be too early to diagnose or may never progress to the clinical stage."[2] This is such an important point! Just because a disease hasn't reached the clinical stage does not mean it isn't affecting your health—and your fertility!

Rather than waiting to treat disease once it has progressed so far, we can consider switching the paradigm to disease prevention and maintenance. We can catch disease processes in the subclinical stage. To do this, it's important to be in tune with your body to notice any early-stage deviations and get regular health checks to monitor any physiological markers of early-stage disease. Preventive maintenance starts *before* disease takes hold. That's exactly what preconception testing is all about.

INFORMED CONSENT

Informed consent is a principle in medicine that a patient must have sufficient information and understanding before making decisions about their medical care. I do not believe that most people are being given appropriate informed consent about their health, especially when it comes to fertility. This entire book, and this chapter specifically, is designed to change that tide. You deserve adequate information about your body so that you can make appropriate decisions about your healthcare that are aligned with your preferences and values today and into the future.

TEST BEFORE YOU TRY

Now that we've talked about *why* to test, let's discuss *what* to test. I've broken down five key areas to test to ensure that your body is in prime condition before you start trying to conceive. As we go through each area, I'm also going to highlight the more common dysregulations that I see.

I recommend preconception testing for any individual or couple who desires to become pregnant in the next twelve months. This will allow you time to correct any abnormalities that might be detected on your tests (which can take at least three to six months and, in some cases, even longer). This way you'll be your healthiest when you're ready to start trying.

For a full list of tests, please go to *www.getpoplin.com*.

Blood Type and Status

- Blood Type: ABO Group, Rh Type
- Complete Blood Count (CBC)
- Ferritin

These tests give you a snapshot of your blood type and the health of your red blood cells, white blood cells, and platelets.

One of the most common (and easily treatable) things that comes up in this category is iron-deficiency anemia. In fact, up to 25 percent of pregnancies experience some form of iron deficiency.[3] This can be easily screened for and addressed beforehand. It's a very standard test that happens in the first trimester of pregnancy. However, once you're in the first trimester of pregnancy, anemia can already have implications not only for your energy levels and fatigue, but also for the growth and development of your baby. Why wait until the first trimester of pregnancy to screen for and address it?

We also know that blood volume increases significantly in pregnancy. If you're on the edge, meaning maybe you're not quite iron deficient yet but you're close, that may increase the likelihood that you'll move into an anemic state once your blood volume changes.

My team and I also see cases where a CBC is normal, but ferritin (iron stores) is low. This is a case where ferritin is a more sensitive marker of iron status than CBC, so changes in ferritin levels will show up earlier than changes in CBC levels. This is another reason that it's important to test a variety of markers—some are more sensitive than others and will show dysregulation earlier.

The more information that we have beforehand, the more we can screen for and address iron-deficiency anemia before going into pregnancy, which will have implications for your ability to have a more seamless experience in pregnancy, as well as for the development of the baby during pregnancy.

Immune Status

- Antibody Screen (females only)
- Antinuclear Antibody (ANA)
- Immunity Status
    - Rubella IgG
    - Varicella IgG
- STI Screening
    - Chlamydia trachomatis
    - Hepatitis B Surface Antigen
    - Hepatitis C Antibody
    - HIV
    - Neisseria gonorrhoeae
    - Reactive Plasma Reagin (syphilis)
    - Trichomonas vaginalis

These tests give you an overview of key immune function markers that could affect fertility and pregnancy, as well as screening for sexually transmitted infections (STIs).

You may be surprised to see an STI screening on a pre-conception test list. I was initially too. However, then I learned that all females are screened for STIs in the first trimester of pregnancy. The question I would ask is this: *If STI status is important to the health of a pregnancy and baby, why are we waiting until a woman is already pregnant to find out? Why wouldn't we screen prior to conception?* Well, that's exactly what I recommend.

It's important to have an STI screening as part of your preconception care because an undiagnosed STI can interfere with your ability to get pregnant or have a healthy pregnancy and baby. For example, chlamydia and gonorrhea, two of the most common sexually transmitted infections, can be asymptomatic and can lead to pelvic inflammatory disease (PID) if left undiagnosed. PID is strongly associated with ectopic pregnancy, infertility, and chronic pelvic pain.[4] Furthermore, Hepatitis B and HIV can both be transmitted from mother to child; early screening and treatment can help prevent this transmission and lower risks of complications for both mom and baby.[5] For male partners as well, it is important to know if you have an STI so that you and your healthcare provider can discuss treatment options; if appropriate care is not received, the STI could be passed to your reproductive partner or future baby, causing complications.

You may not think this is relevant to you, but we have seen cases of positive STI tests that customers were surprised by; they had contracted an STI many years before they met their current partner and were completely asymptomatic. As we discussed in the previous section, many illnesses (including STIs) can be asymptomatic for years! You may have contracted something a while ago and would never have known it. This is exactly why we test!

Rubella and varicella are both infectious diseases that can lead to pregnancy complications and birth defects. Screening for immunity in advance gives you time to get vaccinated if you so choose before conceiving. It is also important for a male partner to get screened for rubella and varicella. Infecting a female partner with rubella during pregnancy can cause miscarriage, stillbirth, and premature birth. It can also cause an infection in your baby called Congenital Rubella Syndrome, which can cause problems with a baby's heart, liver, bones, and spleen. Infecting a female partner with varicella during pregnancy can cause a dangerous form of pneumonia. Varicella infection can also cause an infection in your baby called Congenital Varicella Syndrome.

In addition to STIs and vaccination status, another important thing to screen for is undiagnosed autoimmune conditions; the antinuclear antibody (ANA) test is used to help evaluate a person for autoimmune disorders. Autoimmune conditions are important to screen for because: (a) they are disproportionately present in females, (b) they take a long time to get diagnosed and can wreak all sorts of havoc until then, and (c) they can interfere with your ability to get pregnant, maintain a pregnancy (recurrent miscarriage risk), and have a healthy baby (developmental problems).

I saw undiagnosed autoimmune conditions over and over in my clinical practice—and we are seeing this pattern continue in a disconcertingly large percentage of the customers we test at Poplin. The data here is staggering: 78 percent of autoimmune diagnoses are in females.[6] Moreover, autoimmune conditions are wildly underdiagnosed. In fact, according to a survey by the Autoimmune Diseases

Association, it takes up to 4.6 years and nearly five doctor visits to receive a proper autoimmune-disease diagnosis.[7] Autoimmune conditions can lead to recurrent miscarriage and can also cause problems with the development of the fetus.[8] The antinuclear antibody test is a fairly easy screening test with huge dividends if you happen to catch an autoimmune condition early. If you do end up finding out that you have an autoimmune condition prior to conceiving, it's important that you manage it in partnership with your doctor. The earlier you have the information, the more you can gather resources to address your condition and get the support that you need to make sure that it is well managed prior to pregnancy—and then during pregnancy and beyond.

> *Please note: A positive ANA test alone is not confirmation of autoimmune disease. It is suggestive of autoimmune disease processes but will require follow-up testing and collaboration with your doctor to confirm an autoimmune diagnosis.*
> *Positive ANA results can also be present in ~3–15 percent of healthy individuals.*[9]

Hormone Status

- Reproductive Hormones
  - Anti-Mullerian Hormone (AMH) *(females only)*
  - DHEA Sulfate (DHEAS)
  - Dihydrotestosterone
  - Estradiol (E2)
  - Follicle-Stimulating Hormone (FSH)
  - Luteinizing Hormone (LH)

- Prolactin
- Testosterone—total and free
- Sex Hormone Binding Globulin (SHBG)
- Stress Hormones
  - Cortisol
- Thyroid Function
  - Thyroid-Stimulating Hormone (TSH)
  - Thyroxine (T4)—total and free
  - Triiodothyronine (T3)—total, free, and reverse
  - Thyroglobulin Antibodies
  - Thyroid Peroxidase Antibodies (TPO)

These tests provide a deep dive on key hormones that affect fertility and pregnancy, including sex hormones and stress hormones, as well as a comprehensive thyroid function assessment.

Getting your hormones tested is probably the category that you are most familiar with. These tests look at things that you've probably heard of before when it comes to fertility, like estrogen, testosterone, and follicle-stimulating hormone, as well as things you may not have heard of, like less common hormones and binding proteins.

Getting a full hormone screen, including checking less-commonly discussed hormones and binding proteins, is crucial for getting a full picture of your pre-pregnancy wellness. For example, you may have sufficient hormone levels, but you may have a lot of binding proteins, which essentially inactivates your hormones. In other words, you may have a lot of hormones floating around, but they're not able to do their job well. That's important for us to know because it affects how you would address the issue. Low production of hormones versus high production with mostly inactivated hormones is different. The more nuanced we can get with what's going on, the more places to potentially intervene to optimize your fertility.

An area of concern to be on the lookout for is subclinical hypothyroid disease. A lot of times when doctors look at thyroid function, they only look at thyroid-stimulating hormone (TSH). If you're lucky, they'll look at free T4 as well, and maybe T3. I recommend getting a full thyroid panel, which looks at up to eight different thyroid markers. The reason for that is because even if you have a normal TSH, you could still have thyroid issues, such as abnormal Thyroid Peroxidase or reverse T3 levels. We see this all the time at Poplin. As an example, one test we recently ran had seven normal thyroid levels and only one abnormal result, Thyroglobulin Antibodies. If we had run what most doctors run (TSH only), we never would've caught what was going on. It was a super early disease process, but we were able to identify it at the subclinical stage rather than waiting until overt symptoms started to emerge.

This more in-depth panel is important because TSH is often one of the last things to change. If we're only measuring TSH, we may not be catching earlier stages of thyroid dysfunction. You may be feeling a bit tired, or you may be struggling with your hair thinning out, or you may have issues with constipation. You just may think this is normal, but it might be subclinical hypothyroidism. If we use a broader thyroid panel, we can actually figure out what's going on. Subclinical hypothyroidism can often be addressed through diet and lifestyle interventions. Sometimes, you may need to take thyroid medication. The appropriate treatment plan is something that you should discuss with your doctor. The first step is to see what's going on under the hood!

It's important to address subclinical hypothyroidism before you try to get pregnant because it can affect your ability to get pregnant in the first place as well as affect the development of a baby in utero. Low maternal thyroid hormone levels have been linked to impaired brain development and low IQ in children.[10] For male partners, abnormal thyroid hormone levels can lead to changes in testis function, including semen abnormalities. This is yet another case where the more you know and the earlier you know, the more options you have for intervention.

PRECONCEPTION AND PREGNANCY RANGES

Did you know that the optimal range for TSH is different in the preconception window than for the normal population? True story. This is true for other biomarkers as well. What may be considered acceptable in other life stages may be suboptimal during pregnancy and lead to complications. For optimal outcomes, it is important that your health is more tightly controlled and managed in the preconception and pregnancy windows than at other points in time.

Metabolic Status

- Blood Sugar Management
  - Glucose
  - Hemoglobin A1c (HbA1c)
  - Insulin
- Cholesterol Metabolism
  - Lipid Panel
- Inflammatory Markers
  - Homocysteine
  - High-sensitivity C-reactive Protein (hs-CRP)
- Liver and Kidney Function
  - Alanine Aminotransferase (ALT)
  - Albumin
  - Aspartate Aminotransferase (AST)
  - Bilirubin, total
  - Creatinine

These tests provide a comprehensive look at your metabolic function, including indicators of blood sugar management, cholesterol metabolism, inflammation, and liver function. There are several subcategories within metabolic status. First, let's look at blood sugar function, which is incredibly important when it comes to hormone regulation. Hormones are all intimately connected and interdependent. Too much sugar leads to too much insulin. Too much insulin leads to too much cortisol and too much testosterone. Too much cortisol depletes estrogen and progesterone. Too much insulin and too much cortisol leads to excess body fat. Excess body fat leads to too much estrogen. And the cycle continues. Balanced blood sugar—and hormone levels—is where it's at.

A lot of times, doctors will screen for diabetes, but I frequently see clients who have prediabetes, the stage right before diabetes. Prediabetes indicates that your blood sugar management in your body is dysregulated, which can impact ovulation in females and sperm production in males.[11] We certainly see this disrupted ovulation in cases of polycystic ovary syndrome (PCOS) in females. But you don't have to have diabetes to have anovulatory cycles. In other words, even early stages of blood sugar dysregulation can interfere with ovulation such that you can have periods during which you're not ovulating.

If you know that you have type 2 diabetes or prediabetes, then it will be important to work with your doctor or a nutritionist to either manage or reverse your diabetes prior to getting pregnant. Other indicators of poor blood sugar management are constant sugar cravings, feeling irritable/light-headed if you miss a meal, getting tired after eating, and feeling weak or shaky often. If you suspect that you have issues with blood sugar, it's definitely worth exploring further.

To better understand blood sugar function, I recommend looking at both hemoglobin A1c, which is a traditional measure of your blood sugar, as well as fasting insulin. Fasting insulin is a much earlier measure of what's going on with your blood sugar; it is much more sensitive and will change much earlier than hemoglobin A1c. If we test both markers, we can catch earlier cases of what's going on and therefore can start to make dietary changes that can get your blood sugar status in much better working order.

Second, a lipid panel measures the different types of cholesterol in your body and how they relate to one another. Cholesterol levels naturally increase when you're pregnant and therefore cannot be accurately evaluated during pregnancy. The best way to know what your cholesterol levels are is to measure them before pregnancy. Current studies show that there may be a link between abnormal cholesterol levels and a longer time to conception, an increased risk of preterm birth, and increased cholesterol levels in children.[12]

Next, it's important to look at inflammatory markers. Inflammation may be caused by many conditions, including infection and autoimmune diseases, and has been associated with poor pregnancy outcomes, including lower rates of conception and infertility and increased rates of miscarriage. These outcomes can be driven by inflammatory processes in either reproductive partner. Inflammatory markers are nonspecific (meaning if they are elevated, we don't always know why); however, they are a great jumping-off point to dig deeper to see what might be going on.

Inflammation may sound nebulous, and it can be, but that doesn't make it any less impactful. There is an epidemic of inflammation going on—we eat inflammatory foods and live inflammatory lifestyles. I am seeing this reflected in our clients—up to half of Poplin's customers are showing some sort of inflammation on their test results.

Last but not least, we also want to look at liver function. Liver function is incredibly important because your liver processes all of your hormones. If your liver is congested or operating ineffectively, things can get backed up, causing the stuff that should be excreted to start recirculating in your body. Healthy liver function helps make sure that you're effectively excreting hormones that your body no longer needs.

Nutrient Status

- Folate (Vitamin B9)
- Cobalamin (Vitamin B12)
- Omega-3 and Omega-6 Fatty Acids
- Vitamin D

A test of your nutrient status is an evaluation of critical nutrients responsible for supporting optimal fertility and pregnancy.

The nutrient that you have probably heard the most about is folate. It's incredibly important, certainly for preventing neural tube defects. There are a lot of other unsung heroes when it comes to nutrients in the preconception period, including vitamin B12, Omega-3 and Omega-6 fatty acids, and vitamin D.

I especially want to highlight the importance of vitamin D. Vitamin D has incredibly diverse functions in the body. Vitamin D deficiency can increase maternal risk of gestational diabetes and preeclampsia. It has also been associated with low birthweight, poor skeletal health, impaired brain development, autoimmune disease, obesity, and insulin resistance in babies.[13] Vitamin D levels are easy to measure and fairly easy to address, but it can take up to six months to replete levels, depending on how much of a deficiency you have. Despite the recent attention on vitamin D, we are still seeing the vast majority of individuals running our Poplin panels below optimal levels of vitamin D at the time of this writing.

The only real ways to increase vitamin D levels with reliability are through sun exposure and through supplementation. Unfortunately, there aren't great food sources of vitamin D. The bottom line is that vitamin D is important for health and fertility and is easy to screen for and address when caught early.

I also want to briefly mention omega-3 and omega-6 fats, which are essential fatty acids. An omega-3 and omega-6 fatty acid test measures the levels of these fatty acids in your blood. These levels influence how well your cells function and may play a role in inflammation and fertility. Testing your levels can give you a sense for whether you need to modify your diet or add incremental supplementation. We will discuss this more in Chapter 13.

Across all five of these categories, you want to ensure that any chronic conditions are optimally managed for pregnancy. If you are managing a chronic health condition, such as diabetes, thyroid disease, or autoimmune disease, it is important to work with your doctor to ensure that you are on appropriate medication and appropriate dosages of that medication and that your lab values reflect that your condition is well controlled prior to pregnancy. For example, uncontrolled autoimmune disease can predispose you to miscarriage. Uncontrolled diabetes can increase risks for both mom and baby during pregnancy. See Chapter 8 for more details on working with your doctor to ensure chronic conditions are well managed.

Please note: This is the most current list of testing recommendations as of the writing of this book. My Poplin team and I are constantly monitoring guidelines and evidence to stay up-to-date with the latest science. Accordingly, you may see some changes to these categories over time as preconception care matures and evolves even further.

SCREENING FOR MALES

Males should undergo a similar set of baseline tests because the same imbalances that impact female fertility can also impact male fertility. In addition, unlike with eggs, we can directly measure several markers of sperm function through a semen analysis, including sperm quantity (count + concentration) and sperm quality (motility, morphology, and DNA fragmentation):

- **Sperm count**: The total number of sperm in a particular quantity of semen.

- **Sperm concentration**: How densely packed sperm are within the semen.

- **Sperm motility**: A sperm's ability to move or swim efficiently. According to Legacy, a leading semen analysis company, sperm with high motility move "forward in straight lines or in large circles." Sperm with reduced motility may not be able to move through the female reproductive tract to reach and fertilize the egg.

- **Sperm morphology**: The sperm's structure or shape. A sperm's morphology determines how well it can "swim" toward, penetrate, and fertilize the egg.

- **DNA fragmentation**: Sperm carries DNA which, combined with the DNA in the egg, makes up the full set of DNA of the embryo. DNA fragmentation refers to when the DNA inside the sperm is damaged or broken. According to Legacy, DNA fragmentation correlates to lower fertility and increased risk of recurrent miscarriage.[14]

There are several direct-to-consumer testing companies that offer at-home semen analysis if that's of interest. For semen analysis testing options, go to *www.9monthsisnot enough.com/bookresources*.

ADDITIONAL SCREENING

Above, I've outlined the five main categories of pre-pregnancy wellness that can be tested for on an initial screening test. This is the baseline I recommend for all couples planning to conceive. More specialized testing might be needed depending on your personal circumstances. Other follow-up tests to consider might include:

- Stool analysis
- Adrenal stress index
- Micronutrient testing

- Toxicity/oxidative stress assessment
- Genomics

How to Get Tested

In my experience, many individuals get resistance from their healthcare providers when they request to have comprehensive testing done. This is one of the main reasons that I founded Poplin. If you desire more information about your health, please don't let anyone convince you that it's "unnecessary" to know what's going on inside of your own body. In a lot of cases, it's not your provider's fault—they are operating within a medical system where insurance drives care, not the other way around. There are specialized providers out there, in particular functional or integrative medicine practitioners, who would be more than happy to run comprehensive testing to help you uncover your health status. You may not always know what they will run or what they will charge, but it will almost always be more comprehensive than a traditional doctor's visit. Or you are always welcome to run testing with us at Poplin as a starting point—that way, you know exactly what you are paying for and exactly what you are getting. *See Appendix A for how to order testing.*

CHAPTER SUMMARY

- Fertility is an extension of our overall health, not just our hormones.

- You can't always tell if you're "healthy." Symptoms occur late in the disease process. The only way to know for sure is to test.

- You don't have to wait until you try to conceive to get a sense of your fertility. You can measure your pre-pregnancy wellness in advance.

- Your pre-pregnancy wellness is the state of your health prior to conception, usually the year beforehand.

- Comprehensive pre-pregnancy wellness testing includes blood status, hormone status, immune status, metabolic status, and nutrient status.

- Pre-pregnancy wellness testing is for any individual or couple who desires to become pregnant in the next twelve months.

(7)

TO SCREEN OR NOT TO SCREEN?

Determine whether Genetic Testing Is Right for You and Your Family

A conversation about preconception information gathering would not be complete without addressing genetic carrier screening, a test that can tell you whether you carry genes for certain genetic disorders. Electing to do genetic carrier screening prior to pregnancy allows you to find out your chances of having a child with a genetic disorder.

Unlike pre-pregnancy wellness testing, which I recommend for *everyone planning to conceive*, genetic testing is a personal decision and may or may not be appropriate for you. I want you to be aware of the options so that you can make the best decision for yourself and your family. The goal of genetic screening is to gather information that you can use to guide pregnancy planning based on your personal values.

Genetic carrier screening offers the highest degree of optionality when done *before* pregnancy. Screening before pregnancy allows couples to learn about their reproductive risk and to consider the widest range of reproductive options, including whether or not to become pregnant and whether to use advanced reproductive technologies (e.g., preimplantation genetic diagnosis, use of donor gametes).

WHAT IS A GENETIC DISORDER?

A gene is a small piece of hereditary material (DNA). Genes are instructions that control functions or processes in the body as well as physical traits like eye or hair color. Genetic disorders may be caused by problems with either chromosomes or genes.

WHAT IS GENETIC CARRIER SCREENING?

Genetic carrier screening is focused on identifying genetic disorders caused by mutations in a gene. Most carrier screening is conducted for recessive disorders. For a person to get a recessive disorder, they would need to inherit two recessive genes (one from the biological mother and one from the biological father). If a person has only one gene for a disorder, they are known as a carrier of that genetic disorder. Carriers often do not know that they have a gene for a disorder because they usually do not have symptoms.

According to Invitae, a leading medical genetics company, "Most babies born with a rare genetic condition are born to parents with no family history of that condition."[1]

Carrier screening determines your risk of passing a genetic condition on to your child even if you *do not* present with the condition yourself.

WHO SHOULD CONSIDER GENETIC CARRIER SCREENING?

The American College of Obstetricians and Gynecologists (ACOG) recommends that carrier screening be offered to all *females* who are pregnant or planning to become pregnant. ACOG currently recommends offering all women planning to conceive genetic carrier screening for cystic fibrosis, spinal muscular atrophy, and hemoglobinopathy mutations.[2] Additionally, women in populations deemed at risk should be offered screening for the appropriate mutations (e.g., Tay-Sachs for members of the Ashkenazi Jewish and French Canadian populations, β-thalassemia for African American and Mediterranean populations). Finally, screening for fragile X syndrome should be offered to women with a family history.

However, ACOG is beginning to recommend that *all women be offered expanded carrier screening* given the difficulty in determining ancestral backgrounds and the potential benefit of this information. In their Committee Opinion on Carrier Screening, reaffirmed in 2020, ACOG notes:

In the present multiracial society, it is increasingly difficult to define an individual's ancestry. Therefore, the pretest probability of being a carrier for a specific disorder may not be consistent with previous assumptions

about the prevalence of that disorder in the various eth-
nic and racial groups with which a patient identifies...
this has prompted consideration of panethnic screening...in which carrier screening for a panel of disorders
is offered to all individuals regardless of ethnicity rather
than traditional ethnic-based screening.[3]

WHY CONSIDER GENETIC CARRIER SCREENING BEFORE GETTING PREGNANT?

There are two main goals of carrier screening:

1. Identify asymptomatic couples at risk for having a
   child with an inherited genetic disorder.
2. Give couples actionable information to guide their
   pregnancy planning based on their personal values.

Generally, if a female is found to be a carrier of a specific
condition, her reproductive partner will also be screened.
Having both reproductive partners tested before pregnancy gives you a greater range of options and more time
to make decisions. If both reproductive partners are carriers of the same condition, couples can decide whether or
not to conceive and whether to use advanced reproductive
technologies to reduce the risk of passing on the genetic
disease. Furthermore, "knowledge of carrier status during
pregnancy allows patients to consider prenatal diagnosis;
pregnancy management options; or postnatal management,
such as potential treatment options or availability of palli-
ative care (if appropriate), in the event of an affected fetus.

It also may help decrease the time necessary to diagnose an affected child."[4]

Genetic screening gives you knowledge, which gives you the power to make the right decision for your family. The right option for you may be accepting the risk and choosing to get pregnant. The right option may be to undergo prenatal diagnostic testing with each pregnancy—or choose not to. The right option may be choosing not to have children, adopting, or using a donor egg or sperm. The right option may be to use IVF and preimplantation genetic testing to determine if the fertilized egg has the genetic disorder. Once you have the information, it is up to you to decide.

FAQ: BUT WAIT! HOW DO CARRIER SCREENING TESTS DIFFER FROM PRENATAL DIAGNOSTIC TESTS?

Carrier screening tests assess the risk that a baby will be born with a specific birth defect or genetic disorder. Prenatal diagnostic tests can confirm whether a specific birth defect or genetic disorder is present in the fetus.

For example, prenatal diagnostic tests to detect genetic disorders include amniocentesis and chorionic villus sampling (CVS). Amniocentesis usually is done between fifteen and twenty weeks of pregnancy but can be done up until you give birth. A very thin needle is used to take a small sample of amniotic fluid for testing. The cells are studied to detect the presence of a mutated gene. CVS is done a bit earlier in pregnancy (between ten and thirteen weeks). A small sample of tissue is taken from the placenta, and the cells are checked for the presence of the mutated gene.

You can choose to do both carrier screening and prenatal diagnostic tests, either carrier screening or prenatal diagnostic tests, or neither testing option.

WHAT DOES GENETIC CARRIER SCREENING ENTAIL?

Carrier screening involves testing a sample of blood, saliva, or tissue from the inside of the cheek. There are two possible test results for each gene: positive (you have the gene) or negative (you do not have the gene). Once you have had a carrier screening test for a specific disorder, you do not need to be tested again for that disorder since your genes do not change. Typically, the female partner is tested first (though you may also do concurrent testing of both partners). If test results show that the first partner is not a carrier, then no additional testing is needed. If test results show that the first partner is a carrier, their reproductive partner is then tested.

If you test negative, you are not likely to be a carrier. If your test result is positive, that means you are a carrier for that genetic condition. If your partner tests negative for that genetic condition, the chance of passing on the condition to the fetus is small. However, no screening test checks for every known mutation.

If both parents are carriers for a recessive disorder, then there is a one in four chance that their child will have the disorder (child with disease). There is a one in two chance their child will also be a carrier of that disorder (carrier child).[5]

If both partners are found to be carriers of a genetic condition, genetic counseling will be offered to discuss potential implications and options, including prenatal diagnosis and advanced reproductive technologies.

Please note: Genetic carrier screening is not foolproof. No matter what your test result, there is still a risk of you being a carrier for a genetic disorder. While a negative test result shows that you have a reduced risk of being a carrier, it is not possible for carrier screening to identify all individuals at risk for the screened conditions since not all possible mutations are screened and new mutations may arise.

WHAT ARE MY OPTIONS FOR GENETIC CARRIER SCREENING?

Carrier screening for genetic disorders is completely voluntary. As mentioned previously, ACOG recommends screening all females for cystic fibrosis, spinal muscular atrophy, and hemoglobinopathies. In addition, you may elect to do:

- Targeted carrier screening, where you are tested for disorders based on your ethnicity or family history.

- Expanded carrier screening, where many disorders are tested for at once regardless of race or ethnicity.

Different companies that offer expanded carrier screening create their own lists of disorders they test for and generally focus on severe disorders that impact quality of life from an early age.

Both targeted and expanded carrier screening are considered acceptable strategies for pre-pregnancy and prenatal carrier screening. Expanded carrier screening is the broadest option at this time.

IMPLICATIONS OF GENETIC TESTING ON INSURANCE

One last thing to keep in mind is that genetic testing can affect insurance premiums or eligibility for life or long-term care insurance. While the 2008 federal Genetic Information Nondiscrimination Act makes it illegal for health insurance providers to use genetic information to make decisions about your health insurance eligibility or coverage, this protection does not apply to life, disability, or long-term care insurance.

The information in this chapter is designed to inform you of the potential options; it depends entirely on your personal preference which path to take from here.

If of interest, please see *9monthsisnotenough.com/book resources* for genetic carrier screening providers.

CHAPTER SUMMARY

- Genetic carrier screening is a test that can tell you whether you carry genes for certain genetic disorders. Electing to do genetic carrier screening prior to pregnancy allows you to find out your chances of having a child with a genetic disorder.

- When done before pregnancy, genetic carrier screening offers the highest degree of optionality.

- Genetic carrier screening tests (done before pregnancy) are not the same thing as prenatal diagnostic tests (done during pregnancy).

THE MOST IMPACTFUL DOCTOR'S VISIT OF YOUR LIFE

Schedule a Preconception Visit

"...the preconception visit may be the single most important health-care visit when viewed in the context of its effect on pregnancy."

—PRECONCEPTION HEALTH AND CARE: A LIFE COURSE APPROACH

The birth of a healthy baby to a healthy family depends on a couple's general health before conception as well as on the quality of prenatal and postnatal care. Proper healthcare before pregnancy can ameliorate disease, improve risk status, and help prepare a family for childbearing. Pre-pregnancy or preconception care (PCC) is designed to identify and reduce a couple's reproductive risks *before* conception.

Since the early 1980s, guidelines have recommended preconception care. The American College of Obstetricians and Gynecologists (ACOG) and the Centers for Disease Control (CDC) have both weighed in on the topic with their own sets of preconception care guidelines.[1] In fact, back in 2006, the CDC identified the need for preconception health promotion and care as a critical public health topic and hoped their recommendations would be a starting point to make comprehensive preconception care a standard of care in the United States.[2]

Interesting. What happened since then? And why is no one talking about this?

BARRIERS TO PRECONCEPTION CARE

Despite the clear clinical evidence behind preconception care, less than 20 percent of women report having had a preconception visit prior to pregnancy.[3] There are both physician and patient barriers to effective preconception care.

Most physicians say that they are in favor of the implementation of preconception care but claim that they either don't have enough knowledge/tools to conduct an adequate preconception visit or they don't have enough time to do so effectively. As a result, they just aren't proactively offering this service.

Moreover, few patients know to request a preconception visit.

This huge gap in care is costing us. Together, we are going to start changing that right here and right now. I want to give you the information you need so you can (a) request a preconception visit and (b) come to it prepared to get a full evaluation.

WHAT IS A PRECONCEPTION VISIT?

Most women make an appointment with their care provider once they find out they are pregnant. But did you know that there is such a thing as a preconception visit? Don't worry if not—you're not alone. Most people haven't been told about or offered a preconception visit, which is exactly why we are here!

As a reminder, preconception is the period of time immediately prior to getting pregnant, usually one year beforehand. A preconception visit is the visit with your doctor prior to initiating the process of trying to conceive. The healthcare that you receive from your doctor in the period prior to conceiving is called preconception care (PCC) or pre-pregnancy care.

Your preconception visit is the best time to evaluate all of your fertility KPIs with a medical professional. This will help you evaluate your pre-pregnancy wellness baseline and determine where you need to make changes in your life for the best pregnancy outcomes.

WHY IS A PRECONCEPTION VISIT IMPORTANT?

Preconception healthcare is intended to address the components of health that have been shown to *increase the chances of having a healthy baby*. The goal of a preconception visit is to understand whether you have any risk factors that might affect future pregnancies—and to address them before you start trying to conceive so that you can enter pregnancy in optimal health. Preconception care focuses on taking steps now to protect your health and the health of your baby *in the future.*

Pre-pregnancy care has been shown to lead to better outcomes for both mom and baby. Proper preconception care has two main benefits: it makes it easier to get pregnant, and it increases the likelihood of having a healthy pregnancy and baby. It has been shown to reduce the incidence of fertility, pregnancy, and birth complications, such as babies that are born early or at low birthweight.

Pre-pregnancy care intervenes before the critical period of organogenesis (day seventeen to fifty-six after conception), in contrast to prenatal care, which occurs much later in the development process. The traditional early prenatal visit is *too late* to prevent certain reproductive outcomes such as birth defects resulting from abnormal organ development in trimester one. Further, some interventions that are available prior to conception are not possible once a woman conceives (e.g., certain immunizations, treatment for STIs).

According to the CDC:

> Preconception health is a precious gift to babies. For babies, preconception health means their parents took steps to get healthy before pregnancy. Such babies are less likely to be born early (preterm) or have a low birthweight. They are more likely to be born without birth defects or other disabling conditions. Preconception

health gives babies the best gift of all—the best chance for a healthy start in life.[4]

FAQ: BUT WAIT! CAN'T I JUST HAVE A PRENATAL VISIT?

Prenatal care alone is *just not enough* anymore to ensure healthy babies. Babies are being born too soon, too small, and often, too sick to survive. According to the CDC, "Since 1996, progress in the United States to improve pregnancy outcomes, including low birthweight, premature birth, and infant mortality has slowed."[5] They've determined that "focusing solely on the brief period between prenatal care and childbirth is insufficient... Rather...clinical interventions before pregnancy— in what has come to be known as the 'preconception period'—provide additional opportunities to improve birth outcomes."[6]

This means that prenatal care alone is insufficient to improve maternal and infant outcomes. We need to focus on improving preconception health to drive better outcomes for all. Preconception health expands the point of intervention from solely focusing on pregnancy to a broader lens of that which contributes to health outcomes for mothers and babies—a reproductive couple's health before conception. This also expands the responsibility for a child's health from solely focusing on the female partner's contribution to that of the male reproductive partner as well.

The preconception window is a crucial period for influencing not only pregnancy outcomes, but also future maternal and child health and prevention of long-term conditions. Suffice it to say, the preconception period is really freaking important! In the future, it is likely that the definition of prenatal care will be expanded to include a pre-pregnancy visit as well as ongoing pre-pregnancy interventions, in addition to the currently recommended prenatal care visits. It's coming, but it may be a while. I'm not waiting for that to happen—and it looks like you aren't either. You are way ahead of the curve!

WHAT CAN I EXPECT AT A PRECONCEPTION VISIT WITH MY DOCTOR?

Ideally, preconception care involves more than a single visit to your healthcare provider, but these are some guidelines for what a preconception visit entails. Hopefully this visit can initiate the preconception care conversation. I am outlining these guidelines here so that you can have a reference point for what to discuss with your doctor at a preconception visit. If your doctor doesn't address certain items, I encourage you to bring them up and advocate for yourself! This will ensure that you get the best care possible. Otherwise, you may be missing key information about your reproductive capacity.

A comprehensive preconception visit involves the following evaluations.

Pregnancy Intention

Your provider may inquire about when you plan to start trying to conceive, how many children you would like to have, and how close together you plan to have children ("interpregnancy interval").

PRECONCEPTION TIP

Did you know that the most optimal birth spacing is at least one and a half to two years from the end of one pregnancy to the beginning of the next? Shorter intervals between pregnancies have been shown to increase the risk of pregnancy complications, including preterm birth and low birthweight. Of course, this can be highly individualistic depending on your state of health going into pregnancy, the type of labor and childbirth you experienced, the duration of breastfeeding, and certain other factors. This timeline can also be modifiable depending on how actively you monitor and manage your health postpartum, which is why I advocate for pre-pregnancy wellness testing prior to each pregnancy.

As part of this discussion, your doctor may also inquire about your use of birth control, including the method you are currently using for contraception. This would be a good time to discuss discontinuing birth control, if you are still on it, and to ask for guidance on how and when to stop it.

Reproductive Health History

Your provider may ask about the details of your menstrual cycle over time, including:

• Age of first period (i.e., age of menarche)

- Regularity throughout your life (have you ever lost your period?)
- Flow (duration, how heavy, etc.)
- Symptoms during your period (cramping, bloating, moodiness, etc.)
- Cycle tracking

As a reminder, period symptoms are a good barometer of your overall hormonal health and fertility.

This would also be a good time to make sure that you are up-to-date on your Pap smear, which screens for cervical cancer. You should also plan on discussing your gynecological history, including any previously abnormal Pap smear results, as well as any colposcopy or loop electrosurgical excision procedures (LEEP). When you cover your reproductive health history, your doctor may include a discussion of your sexual history and any sexual challenges (such as pain with intercourse or STI risk factors.)

If relevant, your provider will also discuss your previous pregnancies (elective terminations, miscarriages, preterm births, full-term births, complications, method of delivery). Experiencing an adverse outcome in a previous pregnancy can be an important predictor of future reproductive risk, so it's important to discuss this with your provider to ensure they provide targeted interventions to reduce risks during future pregnancies.

Medical History

You and your provider will discuss your general health history (e.g., chronic conditions, surgeries) along with targeted questions regarding conditions that could affect fertility. Many unfavorable maternal and fetal outcomes are associated with specific preexisting maternal conditions that could be avoided through pre-pregnancy interventions. If not managed well, many chronic conditions (e.g., asthma, hypertension, diabetes, thyroid disorders) can have an adverse effect on pregnancy outcomes, leading to pregnancy loss, infant death, birth defects, or other complications for you and your baby.

Your goal is to work with your doctor to make sure that any medical conditions you have are under control and optimized for pregnancy. In many cases, clinical practice guidelines (CPGs) for preconception care for specific maternal chronic health conditions have been developed by national health professional groups. For example, the American Diabetes Association has developed CPGs that should be followed before pregnancy for women with diabetes; with proper preconception diabetes management, there is a significant reduction in the three-fold increase in prevalence of pregnancy loss and birth defects.[7] The American Association of Clinical Endocrinology has developed CPGs for women with hypothyroidism who are attempting to conceive.[8] For females with hypothyroidism, the required dosages of thyroid medication increase during early pregnancy, and your dosage will need to be adjusted for proper neurologic development of the fetus. These are all items that you can discuss in detail with your provider during the preconception visit.

Medication History

You and your provider will discuss the medications that you use, including over-the-counter, herbal, and prescription drugs and supplements. Prior to your visit, you will want to make a list of any medications or supplements you currently take. It is important to confirm with your doctor that they are fertility and pregnancy safe.

Certain medications are considered teratogenic, meaning they can interfere with fertility and pregnancy health. The list of teratogenic medications includes certain prescription medications, over-the-counter medications, and herbal supplements, so be sure to discuss all the medications and supplements you take with your doctor. The fetus is most susceptible to drug effects during the first trimester of pregnancy, when cells are rapidly dividing and organs are developing. Because of this, *clinical practice guidelines have been developed for women being treated with teratogenic medications to guide the transition to safer medications.* For example, women who have conditions treated with medications that are known to be teratogens (e.g., anticonvulsant or anticoagulant medications) might need to take lower dosages or change prescriptions altogether. Depending on your health condition, certain medications can be swapped for more fertility-friendly options or discontinued altogether for the duration of pregnancy. Please *do not* discontinue any medications on your own without medical advice. Discuss your options with your doctor and make an informed decision from there. Questions to ask include: *Are there safer alternatives to the medications I'm taking? What is the smallest effective dose to treat my condition? If changing medications or dosages, do I have to wait a certain amount of time before I start trying to conceive?*

For males, certain medications (including but not limited to testosterone replacement therapy, steroids, antide-
pressants, chemotherapy drugs, opiates, and NSAIDs) may
have an impact on sperm production and sperm quality.
For a short list of common medications known to interfere
with pregnancy, go to *9monthsisnotenough.com/bookresources.*
No discussion about medications or supplements in
the preconception window would be complete without
addressing prenatal vitamins. Guidelines support the use of
prenatal vitamins prior to conception, so your doctor will
likely encourage you to start taking a prenatal vitamin if
you are planning for an upcoming pregnancy. See Chapter
13 for more details on why this is important.

Family History

Plan on discussing your family history with your provider.
This evaluation will include a discussion of any health
problems that run in your or your reproductive partner's
family (e.g., hypertension, diabetes, thyroid problems, cancer, genetic conditions). This includes grandparents, aunts,
uncles, parents, siblings, children, and cousins. Ideally, you
want to talk to your family in advance to create a family
medical history. You can then share this list with your doctor to identify any additional preventive steps necessary.

Immunization History

Your provider will want to ensure that you're up-to-date
on your vaccinations, particularly for rubella and varicella.
Rubella is a flu-like viral illness. Infection with rubella during
pregnancy can cause miscarriage, stillbirth, and premature

birth. It can also cause an infection in your baby called Congenital Rubella Syndrome. This can cause problems with a baby's heart, liver, bones, and spleen; they can also be born deaf or blind. Varicella, also known as chickenpox, is an infection spread through contact with an infected person's rash or through the air from an infected person's cough or sneeze. Varicella infection during pregnancy can cause complications for the baby such as birth defects, blindness, and seizures.

If you are not immune to rubella or varicella, being vaccinated before pregnancy can help protect you and your baby. Both the rubella and varicella vaccines contain live viruses and therefore cannot be administered during pregnancy. Therefore, it's important to know your status prior to pregnancy in case you do not have immunity and would like to get vaccinated. Some vaccinations will require multiple shots (e.g., varicella). You may also need to wait a certain amount of time after a vaccination before you try to conceive (e.g., twenty-eight days after MMR vaccine).

Social History

As part of your preconception visit, your provider will want to better understand your risk factors and modifiable lifestyle factors. This may include:

- Diet/nutritional status
- Exercise/physical activity
- Body weight
- Environmental and occupational exposures
- Domestic violence, abuse, lack of support
- Alcohol use
- Smoking/recreational drug use

SMOKING

I've addressed most of the items on this list of risk factors in other chapters in the book, so I will keep this interlude brief. Smoking has been shown to affect fertility in many ways.[9] Studies have demonstrated that smoking increases time to conception, affects egg and sperm health, and can cause birth defects.[10]

Smoking cigarettes reduces oxygen levels, constricts placental blood vessels, and strips the body of nutrients. This decreases oxygen capacity and nutrient stores. The chemicals from cigarette smoke also affect every stage of the reproductive cycle and influence hormone production for both females and males. The oxidative stress caused by smoking leads to damaged DNA in the eggs and sperm and causes inflammation in the uterus, which can inhibit implantation and impair the quality of the uterine lining.

Smoking during pregnancy has been linked to increased risk of ectopic pregnancy (embryo implants outside of the uterus, most commonly in the fallopian tube), miscarriage, low birthweight, premature birth, and birth defects.

If you've still been holding onto this habit and would like to quit, the preconception period is the perfect time to make it happen. The moment you stop smoking, your body can start getting to work on detoxifying and repairing any damage.

Physical Exam

Your provider will likely conduct some sort of physical exam, especially if you haven't had one in over a year. During your physical exam, they will assess your vital signs, including blood pressure, heart rate, and weight. It's important to know these vitals prior to pregnancy because they will change during pregnancy, and providers want to have a baseline.

PRECONCEPTION TIP

Schedule a dental cleaning if you haven't had one in the last six months. All females should get a dental checkup prior to trying to conceive. Studies have shown that having poor dental health can not only affect fertility but can also lead to pregnancy complications for both mom and baby. According to the CDC, dental caries (early stages of tooth decay) and other oral diseases are both common (found in over 80 percent of women aged twenty to thirty-nine years) and associated with complications for women and infants.[11]

What Does Oral Health Have to Do with Fertility?

You're probably familiar with the microbiome of your gut—trillions of microbes (i.e., bacteria, fungi, viruses, etc.) that live in your GI tract. You also have an oral microbiome. This makes sense when you think about the fact that your mouth is really the beginning of your GI tract. Your oral microbiome is influenced by many factors, including your diet, daily brushing and flossing habits, and regular dental cleanings. An imbalance in the oral microbiome can result in things like gum disease and inflammation in the mouth.

Studies have shown that periodontitis (or gum disease) is associated with increased time to conception and increased miscarriage risk. Researchers believe that this connection could be due to low-grade systemic inflammation caused by periodontitis or from bacteria from the gums making their way to amniotic fluid, causing an immune response.[12] It's an immune and inflammatory cascade.

What is the Connection between Oral Health and Pregnancy Complications?

Pregnancy is notoriously hard on your oral health. The increase in hormones during pregnancy can increase your chances of developing gingivitis, which is an early stage of periodontitis (PD). Changes in diet (e.g., eating more sugar or refined carbohydrates due to food aversions) and increased acidity in the mouth due to morning sickness can also lead to cavities. A woman's gums also become softer and more vascular during pregnancy, which makes them more vulnerable to inflammation and infection. In addition, there are several pregnancy complications that are associated with PD, including higher rates of preeclampsia in mom and premature labor and low birthweight for baby.[13] There are also links between a mother's oral health and her baby's risk for dental caries; ideally, you want to reduce the probability of this mother-to-child transmission of cariogenic bacteria. Going into pregnancy with the best oral health possible can help minimize these problems.

If you've been holding off, it is also important to get any dental procedures prior to pregnancy (e.g., cavities filled, root canals, etc.). This is because it is generally unsafe and therefore inadvisable to undergo major dental work during pregnancy. There are a host of potential dangers to the baby from X-rays, drugs, and the stress of drilling. If you have a dental issue present prior to pregnancy, you don't want to have to wait nine-plus months for it to progress before you can have it taken care of. A dental exam in the preconception period can inform you of any issues that need to be addressed so that you can clear them up with plenty of time before you get pregnant.

This word of caution also applies to males—periodontitis can be a source of chronic infection and inflammation, impacting overall health and sperm health.

Bottom line: If you've fallen behind on scheduling your twice-yearly dental cleaning, now's the time to make the call. The preconception period is the perfect time to reprioritize oral health, including daily brushing and flossing and visiting the dentist every six months.

Lab Work

We did a deep dive on lab work in Chapter 6, so I will keep this section fairly brief.

The unfortunate reality is that most doctors will not run any preconception labs unless you specifically ask them to. Even if you ask them, they may not be familiar enough with the guidelines to know which tests to run. This is where it's important for you to advocate for yourself.

The essential preconception tests based on the most recent guidelines are: ABO Group/Rh Type, Antibody screen, Complete Blood Count (CBC), immunity testing (Rubella, Varicella), and STI testing (Hepatitis B, Hepatitis C, HIV, Syphilis). However, as I outlined previously, this is only a fraction of your overall pre-pregnancy wellness, and I would consider it to be the bare minimum.

I would like to say that you can ask your physician to run the full list of tests in Chapter 6, but in the years that I've been practicing, I've never seen it happen successfully. Even if you somehow were able to make it happen, it would likely be thousands of dollars out of pocket. This is precisely the reason that I founded Poplin.

If you've run lab testing on your own, your preconception visit would be a good time to share your results with your doctor and discuss any necessary interventions. Despite the fact that doctors are unlikely to run as broad a panel of tests as we do at Poplin, they usually will engage once you have lab work in hand, especially with any abnormal findings. This is one of the reasons that it can be helpful to run lab work in advance: it can also allow the time spent with your doctor to be more focused and directed.

ARE PRECONCEPTION VISITS ONLY FOR FEMALES?

"Preconception health is important for men, too."

—CDC

The same areas that we evaluate for females should also be evaluated for males because they can impact overall health as well as fertility.

For example, studies show that men who drink a lot, smoke, or use drugs can have problems with their sperm. These can cause problems with getting pregnant. Male partners can improve their own reproductive health and overall health by limiting alcohol, quitting smoking or illegal drug use, making healthy food choices, and reducing stress.

It is also important to screen for and treat sexually transmitted infections (STIs) to ensure that infections are not passed to female partners—and babies.

Male reproductive partners: I encourage you to talk to your doctor about your health, your family health history, and any medicines you use. Certain medications, such as PPIs and SSRIs, may impact sperm quality.[14] These are some of the most commonly prescribed drugs in the US, so it is up to you to bring this up and discuss it with your doctor if you are planning to conceive soon.

Phew. That's a lot to cover! Given that the average doctor's appointment is around fifteen to twenty minutes, it can be challenging to cover all these topics in depth. For this reason, it's important that you come prepared and, if possible, that you seek out a provider who can spend the requisite time with you to do proper planning and troubleshooting.

At the end of your preconception visit, you should walk away with a plan of action for how to improve your health in order to increase the chances of getting pregnant and having a healthy baby, including but not limited to lifestyle behaviors to modify, medications or supplements to add/change/

discontinue, environmental exposures to modify, referrals to other specialists, and any other health issues to address.

DON'T FORGET ABOUT INSURANCE!

Getting your body in baby-ready shape is a big piece of the preconception puzzle. Another area to address is administrative planning, including health insurance, life insurance, and disability insurance. This is not my area of expertise, but it felt remiss not to mention it, so I will keep this brief and highlight a few important points to keep in mind. I encourage you to work more closely with someone who can help guide you through these important tasks.

Health Insurance

Pregnancy is a time filled with lots of doctor visits along with a higher potential for medical complications that may require additional care. If you are thinking about starting a family, now is the time to check your insurance policy and make sure that it has the coverage you need and want. Here's why: getting pregnant is not a qualifying life event for a special enrollment period in the marketplace. (Interestingly, giving birth and fostering/adopting a child are considered qualifying life events.) The health plan you have when you conceive is the health plan that you will have throughout pregnancy unless you happen to have another qualifying life event or the open enrollment period is coming up. This is one of the many reasons it's important to start preconception planning early!

Life and Disability Insurance

Experts recommend that females get both disability and life insurance *before* they try to get pregnant. Males can wait until they have a dependent. Here's why: certain health conditions or complications can occur during pregnancy (e.g., gestational diabetes, preeclampsia, recurrent miscarriage). For life insurance, these conditions/complications can affect life insurance premiums significantly for years to come. For disability insurance, carriers can refuse to cover disability requests if you have certain medical history, including complications that can occur during preconception, pregnancy, and postpartum. For these reasons, it's ideal to have these insurance policies in place *before* you are pregnant.

CHAPTER SUMMARY

- There have been guidelines on proper preconception care for over forty years, but only 20 percent of women report having had a preconception care visit before pregnancy.

- The goal of a preconception visit is to understand whether you have any risk factors that might affect future pregnancies—and address them beforehand.

- A preconception visit usually consists of ob-gyn history, medical history, medication history, immunization history, family history, social history, and a physical exam.

- You should walk away from a preconception visit with a clear plan of action for how to improve your health in order to increase the chances of getting pregnant and having a healthy baby.

INTERVENTIONS STAGE

How Can You Proactively Address the Top Fertility Blockers?

Now that you have assessed your pre-pregnancy baseline and conducted your preconception visit, you know what you are working with! In addition to the specific actions that you've identified from your discussion with your doctor, there are general actions that are beneficial for anyone planning to conceive. In this next section, we are going to discuss how to address the most common fertility blockers. As we discussed in Section 1, our natural essence is fertile, but our lifestyle and environment have erected barriers to this natural state. It is our job to systematically identify and remove those barriers.

As we go through this next section, it is important to keep in mind that health is a skill that can be learned and refined over time. You may feel like you are well on your way, or you may feel like you have a long way to go. You may feel like some categories come more easily than others. Regardless of your starting point, you can improve your health skill level. I am still improving mine each and every day, learning and implementing new practices to do just a bit better.

IT'S NOT YOU; IT'S YOUR ENVIRONMENT
Optimize Your Environment for Fertility

STATUS CHECK

To get a check on how your detoxification function is working, we can look at a few different markers. If any of these markers is out of balance, it might be a sign that your toxic load is high.

- Metabolic Status
  - Liver Function (Albumin, ALT, AST)
  - Inflammatory Markers (Homocysteine, hs-CRP)
- Hormone Status
  - Reproductive Hormones (Estradiol)

Liver function markers will give us a sense for how your liver is operating. Because the liver is a primary detoxification organ, it's important that

---

it's operating in tip-top shape. A high toxin load puts stress on the body, and that can show up as increased inflammation. Lastly, did you know that estrogen can become toxic at high levels? Yes, it has been shown to play a role in estrogen-sensitive cancers, for example. We are exposed to many different forms of estrogen (e.g., phytoestrogens, xenoestrogens) in our daily life. Looking at your overall estrogen level can give you a sense for whether your estrogen levels might be too high, potentially due to external exposures.

According to Dr. David L. Katz:

You don't need to be gluttonous to overeat or lazy to underexercise and gain weight in the modern world; you simply need to live in the modern world, which is why obesity and chronic diseases are not exceptions— they are now the norm. There's a place for both personal responsibility and public policy in fixing what ails our collective health. While you're waiting for the world to change, it is possible to steer the course of your own and your family's health in a better direction.[1]

Let me state this clearly and unequivocally: our environment is infertile-genic. Just like our environment has been classified as obesogenic (i.e., predisposes us to weight gain), so it is infertile-genic (i.e., predisposes us to infertility).[2] Managing your environment is one of the missing links in all of health—and fertility.

Suffice it to say, the deck is not stacked in your favor. But you've already made it this far in the book, so I can see that you're committed. You don't need to just accept the cards we've all been dealt; you can reshuffle the deck and stack it in your favor. Engineer your environment to beat the odds. This entire chapter is dedicated to teaching you how.

At a high level, the punch line, according to the CDC, is this: "Avoid harmful chemicals, environmental contaminants, and other toxic substances...around the home and in the workplace. These substances can hurt the reproductive systems of men and women. They can make it more difficult to get pregnant."[3]

Minimizing your exposure to environmental toxins that can harm fertility is one of the best steps you can take to increase your chances of getting pregnant and having a healthy baby.

TOXICITY AND FERTILITY

We all have a toxic body burden. For some of us, that burden is quite heavy. For others, not as much. If you suspect that your toxic burden is an issue, I encourage you to consider doing a clinical detox at least nine months prior to conceiving (ideally longer if your toxic burden is substantial) with the support of a skilled practitioner. To be clear, I'm not talking about a juice cleanse.

Why do we detox *before* getting pregnant?

Two main reasons:

1. **Toxicity can interfere with fertility, leading to problems getting pregnant.** A body overloaded

with toxins will have a harder time reproducing. In its infinite wisdom, your body will shut down reproduction any time it perceives the environment into which it will bring a child to be either unsafe or unstable. A toxic body indicates a toxic environment, and your body shuts down reproductive function to protect both you and your future baby.

2. **Toxic compounds can pass from mom to baby, leading to problems having a healthy baby.** A study by the Environmental Working Group (EWG) identified over two hundred industrial compounds and pollutants in samples of newborn babies' umbilical cord blood.[4] This means that some percentage of a mother's toxic body burden is being transferred to her baby. Because of this, detoxing prior to pregnancy can help minimize the transfer of toxic compounds from mama to baby.

Many chemicals persist in your body even after the initial exposure. If you wait until you are already pregnant, you likely will not be able to get rid of all of the chemicals stored in your body. As a result, these chemicals can cross the placenta and even show up in your breast milk once the baby is born, as the EWG study showed. In addition, many chemicals bioaccumulate, meaning they build up in your system over time. Certain substances, like polychlorinated biphenyls (PCBs), get sequestered in your body fat; others, like mercury, get concentrated in specific organs. You may require fat loss or targeted detoxification protocols to liberate these compounds from your body. These things take time!

WHAT ARE TOXINS, AND WHERE DO THEY COME FROM?

Toxin sounds far more dramatic than it needs to. At the simplest level, a toxin is anything physical, chemical, or biological that produces an adverse effect. Toxins impair the proper functioning of your organs by creating a cascade of negative reactions throughout the body. In addition to disrupting the normal flow and function of your organ systems, all toxins create oxidative damage that can impair mitochondrial function. In order to maintain good egg and sperm health, you also need to maintain good mitochondrial health.

Toxins can come from the external environment (exogenous), or they can be generated internally within your body (endogenous). The most prevalent external toxins come from air (e.g., solvents, mold), water (e.g., heavy metals, medications), food (e.g., pesticides, food additives, hormones), personal care products (e.g., endocrine disruptors in shampoo, lotion, makeup, etc.), and home care products (e.g., cleaning chemicals). The most common internal toxins (yes, there are such things as toxins produced internally!) come from metabolic processes, such as bacterial byproducts and oxidative stress.

Unfortunately, most of us are unwittingly exposed to more toxins than we ever considered in the course of daily living. Our bodies have trouble eliminating substances they were never designed to process in the first place. As a reminder from Chapter 3, over twenty thousand chemicals have been added to the Toxic Substances Control Act Inventory since its inception in 1975, and our food supply has changed more in the last fifty years than it did in the previous ten thousand.[5] Our body is being exposed to many new and unfamiliar compounds; these compounds are accumulating at an increasing pace and at a faster rate than our bodies can eliminate them.

HOW DO TOXIN EXPOSURES AFFECT FERTILITY?

Toxins can affect fertility directly or indirectly. First, we will discuss the direct impact of environmental chemicals on fertility through endocrine-disrupting chemicals.

The endocrine system helps regulate your body's development and supports optimal functioning. It is composed of glands and organs that produce, store, and secrete different hormones. As the name implies, endocrine-disrupting chemicals (EDCs) are substances that interfere with the proper functioning of the endocrine system. EDCs can come through the air we breathe, the food we eat, the water we drink, and through our skin from the products we use.

Examples of how EDCs can interfere with our hormones include:

- Mimicking our hormones and tricking our body into thinking that they are hormones
- Blocking our natural hormones from doing their job

- Increasing or decreasing hormone levels in our body by affecting how they are made, broken down, or stored
- Changing how sensitive our bodies are to different hormones

This means that EDCs can interfere with the proper production and function of our hormone levels. This interference can cause a host of downstream effects, including "alterations in sperm quality and fertility, abnormalities in sex organs, endometriosis, early puberty, altered nervous system function, immune function, certain cancers, respiratory problems, metabolic issues, diabetes, obesity, cardiovascular problems, growth, neurological and learning disabilities, and more."[6]

In other words, EDCs are "reproductive toxins," meaning they are destructive to our reproductive system and can interfere with menstrual cycles, egg/sperm development, and fertility, impacting time to conception, miscarriage risk, and pregnancy outcomes.

As of this writing, approximately one thousand chemicals believed to have endocrine-disrupting properties have been identified. (For the most current list of endocrine disruptors, see *9monthsisnotenough.com/bookresources*.[7]) I suspect that there are many more still to be identified. Common EDCs include pesticides (e.g., dichlorodiphenyltrichloroethane or DDT, atrazine, glyphosate), industrial solvents and byproducts (e.g., PCBs, dioxins), plastics and food storage materials (e.g., bisphenol A or BPA, phthalates), electronics and building materials (e.g., brominated flame retardants,

PCBs), personal care products (e.g., phthalates, parabens), and textiles/clothing (e.g., perfluorochemicals).

To put it bluntly, according to the Endocrine Society:

> The increased prevalence over the past 50 years of hormone-sensitive cancers (e.g., breast, prostate), compromised fertility, early puberty, decreased sperm counts, genital malformations, and unbalanced sex ratios... are at least partially attributable to increased chemical abundance and exposures.[8]

Let's dive in deeper on the impacts of EDCs related to fertility.

Damage to a Female's Eggs

Exposure to endocrine disruptors can interfere with hormone systems and harm developing eggs, which can increase miscarriage risk and delay time to pregnancy. For example, exposure to harmful chemicals in critical stages of egg and sperm development can interfere with proper development.[9] Phthalates can mimic estrogen and bind to estrogen receptors, potentially affecting estrogen production and consequently interfering with growth of ovarian follicles.[10] BPA has been linked with reduced egg quality in patients seeking fertility treatment. Other estrogenic EDCs have been associated with uterine fibroids, ovarian dysfunction, and subfertility.[11] In addition, exposure to endocrine-disrupting chemicals increases oxidative stress, which has been shown to play a role in the etiology of ovarian aging.[12] Many endocrine disruptors can interfere with normal menstrual cycles and ovulation and compromise egg quality, thus having profound impacts on fertility.

Damage to a Male's Sperm

Many of the same challenges apply to sperm. EDCs interfere with hormone metabolism, transport, and excretion, and they disrupt sperm development and increase oxidative stress. This can cause problems maintaining proper hormone levels, including androgens such as DHEA and testosterone. This results in impaired sperm production and lower sperm counts, poor morphology, and increased DNA fragmentation.[13] For example, PCB and phthalate exposure have been shown to impact sperm quality, even at low doses.[14]

Imbalanced Hormones and
Irregular Menstrual Cycles

As a reminder, hormones abide by the Goldilocks phenomenon: not too much, not too little, right in the middle. According to the CDC, exposure to certain chemicals may disrupt the balance between the brain, pituitary gland, and ovaries, creating an imbalance of estrogen and progesterone and interfering with regular ovulation and menstrual cycles.[15] An overabundance of one hormone in proportion to another (such as too much estrogen in comparison to progesterone) can wreak havoc on menstrual cycles, causing a host of premenstrual symptoms (such as heavy bleeding or breast tenderness), as well as disrupting ovulation and impairing fertility.

Interference with Fetal Development

It appears that there are windows of susceptibility for EDC exposure; some of the most susceptible periods are in utero and in early postnatal life. Certain EDC exposures can be toxic to developing babies during pregnancy. For example, certain EDCs have been shown to increase the risk of birth defects by increasing the risk of chromosomally abnormal eggs or sperm.[16]

It is important to note that reproductive hazards do not affect every person similarly. Your susceptibility relies on: (1) type of exposure, (2) route and magnitude of exposure (i.e., how you were exposed, how much you were exposed to), and (3) your personal health and susceptibility (e.g., age, immune status, stage of pregnancy). Furthermore, exposures to the same hazard could result in different outcomes, depending on the timing. The CDC notes:

> Exposure to a hazard could block ovulation and pregnancy only at specific times of the menstrual cycle. Exposure during the first 3 months of pregnancy might cause a birth defect or a miscarriage. Exposure during the last 6 months of pregnancy could slow the baby's growth, affect its brain development, or cause premature labor.[17]

A variety of toxic exposures can also indirectly affect your fertility. For example, mold exposure can put strain on your immune system, which can make you more susceptible to infection, allergic reactions, asthma, and mood disorders, all of which can impact your ability to get pregnant. Many environmental chemicals/compounds can increase oxidative stress and inflammation in the body, which can impair egg and sperm quality.

HOW CAN I EFFECTIVELY DETOXIFY?

Okay, that previous part was pretty heavy. But now that you understand how profound and far-reaching the effects of EDCs are, let's talk about what you can do about it.

The goal of detoxification is to remove any obstructions to flow or function and open the channels of elimination. In an ideal world, a strong detoxification system encourages any toxins that inevitably get into your system to exit quickly without leaving too much of a trace.

PRECONCEPTION TIP

It is not advised to detox *during* pregnancy. During the detox process, many compounds become more potent and harmful prior to being excreted from the body, so you want to take it slowly. It takes quite some time for your blood levels to normalize again after slowly releasing these toxins from your body, and you wouldn't want your baby to be exposed to such powerful, detrimental substances for any period of time. It's just too risky.

It is not practical to remove all toxic exposures. We encounter toxins all day, every day. Our goal is to help our body to process them effectively. To that end, there are two main goals of an effective detoxification regimen:

1. Reduce toxic exposure.
2. Increase detoxification capacity.

Reduce Toxic Exposure

The first step is to reduce the number of toxins that you're exposed to on a daily basis. Luckily, the majority of toxins are nonpersistent. In other words, if you stop the exposure to the toxin, it will be eliminated from the body.

Let's take a look at the five major sources of daily toxin exposures that are within your control.

Air

When we think about air quality, we often think about outdoor air. However, indoor air quality is even more important. Many nonpersistent toxicants are airborne, but we are exposed to them mainly from indoor air—at work and at home.

According to the National Human Activity Pattern Survey, humans spend 90 percent of their time indoors.[18] As a result, indoor air quality has a significant influence on human health. Moreover, it has been shown that pollutant levels are, on average, two to five times higher indoors than outdoors.

Indoor pollutants can be classified into three main categories:

1. **Combustion byproducts**: Includes gases and particles released by heating or cooking appliances that rely on combustion, such as carbon monoxide

2. **Volatile Organic Compounds (VOCs)**: Includes a broad category of substances found in sources such as construction materials and cleaning and personal care products

3. **Allergens and asthma triggers**: Includes dust, pollen, mites, pet dander, and mold

There are a variety of methods to improve indoor air quality, but they all focus on two primary goals: reducing the concentration of air pollutants and maintaining humidity within appropriate levels.

Here are a few suggestions to get you started, all courtesy of foobot, an indoor air quality monitoring device:

- **Always use an exhaust hood during and after cooking to ventilate air.** Just because you can't smell the odor of food after cooking doesn't mean pollutants aren't still there. Air-quality monitors have shown that pollution levels can remain high for up to eight hours after cooking.

- **Open windows daily.** According to the EPA, indoor levels of pollutants may be two to five times higher than outdoor levels.[19] Opening windows is a simple, cheap, and quick way to get rid of harmful substances that accumulate in your home. There are only a few instances when opening the windows is not recommended (e.g., times of heavy traffic, times when there is a high concentration of pollen outside).

- **Clean the filters in your HVAC equipment frequently.** HVAC equipment should come equipped with filters, but they lose effectiveness once they become saturated with dust and other pollutants. Congested filters are detrimental for air quality because they restrict airflow and require more energy to push air through the congested filter. This logic also applies to having your air ducts cleaned, ideally every three to five years. If the ducts are dirty, fresh air will be polluted along the way and subsequently distributed throughout your home. A quick way to tell whether your vents need maintenance is to put a piece of paper on a return vent; if it doesn't stick, it's time to get your ducts cleaned.

- **Reduce sources of VOCs from the products you use.** First, it is prudent to familiarize yourself with what VOCs are and where they come from in order to avoid products that mention them in the label (see the sections below on personal and home care products). A good place to start is minimizing the use of scented candles and synthetic fragrances, which release lots of VOCs. Use candles/incense/ room fragrance sparingly, and ventilate well while using. Try to pick natural alternatives and minimize the use of aerosol sprays whenever possible.

- **Use doormats for all entrances.** A considerable number of air pollutants are brought indoors by shoes. Doormats are a quick and effective solution that minimizes the number of pollutants that make it inside your home.

- **Keep humidity within the recommended range.** The American Society of Heating, Refrigerating and Air-Conditioning Engineers (ASHRAE), an organization dedicated to building systems, energy efficiency, indoor air quality, refrigeration, and sustainability, recommends relative humidity levels of 30–60 percent for optimal health and comfort.[20] Both low- and high-humidity levels can cause problems. Low-humidity levels can lead to eye, skin, and nose irritation; high levels can stimulate the growth of unwelcome entities (e.g., bacteria, dust mites, mold, fungi).

- **Use plants to improve indoor air quality.** Did you know that you can enhance indoor air quality with plants? All plants absorb carbon dioxide and emit fresh oxygen. Certain plants have also been shown to absorb VOCs and act as a de facto air filter. These include snake plants, aloe vera, spider plants, areca palm, and rubber plants.

- **Get a high-quality air filter.** Despite the best habits, VOCs are going to be part of an indoor environment. High-quality air filters can be a great addition to keeping the home environment clean and clear.

Water

We are exposed to a host of compounds through our water. Here's what was found in the local New Jersey borough where I grew up, according to their annual water report:

> The sources of drinking water…include rivers, lakes, streams, ponds, reservoirs, springs, and wells. As water travels over the surface of the land or through the ground, it dissolves naturally-occurring minerals and, in some cases, radioactive material, and can pick up substances resulting from the presence of animals or from human activity.[21]

Contaminants in the water may include any of the following:

- **Microbial contaminants (e.g., viruses, bacteria)**, which can come from sewage treatment plants, septic systems, livestock operations, or wildlife

- **Inorganic contaminants (e.g., salts, metals)**, which can be naturally occurring or result from urban stormwater runoff, wastewater discharges, oil and gas production, mining, or farming

- **Pesticides and herbicides,** which can come from a variety of sources such as agriculture or residential use

- **Organic chemical contaminants (e.g., synthetic and volatile organic chemicals),** which are byproducts of industrial processes or can come from gas stations, urban stormwater runoff, and septic systems

- **Radioactive contaminants,** which can be naturally occurring or the result of oil and gas production and mining

Yikes! That's a disconcerting amount of icky stuff in our water!

The annual report continues:

> Some people may be more vulnerable to contaminants in drinking water than the general population. Immuno-compromised persons such as persons with cancer undergoing chemotherapy, persons who have undergone organ transplants, people with HIV/AIDS or other immune system disorders, some elderly, and infants can be particularly at risk from infections.[22]

Did you know that pregnancy is technically also an immunocompromised state? That's why vigilance in and around that time period is super important—for both you and baby.

So what can you do about this? First, you can test your local water so you know what you're dealing with. For information on how to test your local water, see *9month-sisnotenough.com/bookresources*. Next, you can improve the quality of the water that you are exposed to by getting a high-quality water filter for both drinking and shower water. Everyone forgets about the shower filter, but not you! What goes on your body also goes in your body. Whichever option you choose, the goal is to remove the bad stuff (toxic contaminants) and keep the good stuff (minerals) in the water.

Food

Choosing organic fruits and vegetables and organic, pastured animal products whenever possible will reduce your exposure to unnecessary hormones and pesticides. We'll cover nutrition and diet more thoroughly in Chapter 12.

Personal Care Products

A survey run by the Environmental Working Group (EWG) revealed that the average woman uses twelve personal care products (containing 168 unique chemicals) on a daily basis.[23] Because females tend to use a disproportionately higher number of personal care products (e.g., perfume, makeup, lotion, nail polish), a female's toxin load is usually much more substantial than her male counterparts.

Here's where the problem comes in: unlike with drugs, cosmetic products and ingredients (except color additives) do not need FDA premarket approval prior to being released to the public.[24] This means that there is *no safety testing* required before a product is offered for sale to the public. There is also no recall ability. Once a chemical goes onto the market, it can't be pulled from shelves unless it's "proven" to cause harm—and the bar for proof is very high. So it's easy to get products on shelves and hard to get them off. Moreover, cosmetics regulations have not materially changed since 1938 when the Federal Food, Drug, and Cosmetic Act was put into effect.[25] If it is not obvious at this point, there is entirely too little regulation in this area for optimal health.

In fact, many of the ingredients allowed in US products (such as benzene and diethanolamine) have been banned in other countries. For example, the European Union has restricted or banned over two thousand harmful ingredients from personal care products, and Canada has prohibited or restricted several hundred ingredients as well.[26] In the US, the FDA originally banned eleven ingredients and has added another handful of ingredients since (including plastic microbeads and triclosan and triclocarban).[27] However, we are quite far behind other nations.

Personal care product companies may have different formulations of their products depending on local regulations. For example, the formulation of a baby shampoo from the same company can be different in Canada, France, and the United States. This suggests that personal care companies often have the capability and know-how to make safer products across all countries they serve, but they may not unless they are mandated to do so—or customers start demanding it.

Our current regulatory approach in the US suggests an "innocent until proven guilty" theory with each new ingredient. That approach makes sense when it comes to legal trials, but not when it comes to our collective health. Unfortunately, many of these chemicals have been shown to affect both our health and our fertility. We are running a huge epidemiological study that none of us knowingly opted in to.

Until regulations catch up, consumers bear the burden of selecting nontoxic products themselves. I suggest checking out the Environmental Working Group's Skin Deep database to search for cosmetics and find out how yours stack up.[28] It is up to you to proactively safeguard your health and the health of your family, especially until we have more robust regulation on this topic. The Personal Care Products Safety Act is one such regulatory proposal introduced in 2015, but we are still awaiting further action years later. In the meantime, it is up to you to be an informed consumer with anything that goes on or around your body.

Home Care Products

Many of the same tenets apply to home care products as personal care products. Anything that goes in, on, or around your body can be absorbed—through the air you breathe and your skin—and can therefore impact your hormones.

Cleaning products with harsh chemicals may eliminate viruses, fungi, and bacteria but the vapors from these cleaning products remain in the air long after use. More wise words from our friends at foobot, a company that produces indoor air-quality monitors: "A gentle and regular cleaning is better for the air and your health...airing the room out is as important as cleaning it...remember that cleanliness has no smell."

Selecting more natural alternatives here is your best bet. This includes not only cleaning supplies but also things like cookware, utensils, and food storage containers, which can leach toxins into your food.

I know that this can seem daunting. Take your time. I've found that my clients are most successful when they break the task down and tackle upgrades room by room (e.g., bathroom, kitchen, laundry room, bedroom). Managing these five areas alone will provide huge strides in reducing your daily toxin load.

Increase Your Detoxification Capacity

Now that we've discussed how to minimize the toxins coming in, we can move on to address how we can increase the toxins going out.

FAQ: BUT WAIT! DOESN'T MY BODY NATURALLY DETOXIFY ITSELF?

Yes. If you were living in a cave with a pristine water source nearby and getting nine hours of sleep per night and meditating daily, then maybe you wouldn't need additional detox support. But I'm going to guess that's not the case for most of us. Given our modern environment, we are exposed to more chemicals than our bodies can process. As a result, most of us need to take extra steps to up-regulate the function of our detox organs to adequately handle the increased toxin load we are exposed to on a daily basis.

We eliminate toxins from our body through urine, stool, sweat, and breath. In order to get the full benefit of our detoxification plan, we need to improve the function of our detox organs—liver, lungs, skin, colon, kidney (and lymph system). Each of these organs works to eliminate excess waste that's produced from natural metabolic processes (endogenous toxins) as well as from our exposures of daily living (exogenous toxins). To improve their function, we need to give our organs what they need (in the form of nutrients and circulation) and take away what they don't (in the form of toxins and stagnation). For females, this also includes supporting the gentle cleansing of the uterus to dispel any stagnant blood, improve circulation, and fortify uterine tissue for implantation.

While we aim to support all of your detox organs, the real superstar of the show is the liver. Without a healthy liver, there is no hormonal balance. This is where I tell you to go ahead and love up on your liver!

The components of detoxification support include a variety of diet, supplementation, and lifestyle practices, such as:

- Supporting nutrition (through diet, supplementation)
- Supporting elimination (through hydration, diet, supplementation, enema/colon hydrotherapy)
- Supporting sweating (through exercise, sauna)
- Supporting circulation (through hydration, abdominal massage, exercise/movement, hot/cold contrast showers)
- Supporting lymphatic drainage (through skin brushing, jumping/rebounding)

I'll highlight each of these areas briefly, though many of them overlap.

Supporting Nutrition

Your body naturally detoxifies itself. We want to support the body in doing so by providing the nutrients it requires to move the body through the phases of detoxification. Phase 1 detoxification requires many vitamins (such as B vitamins and vitamin C), minerals (such as calcium), and antioxidants (such as N-Acetyl Cysteine). Phase 2 detoxification requires amino acids (such as glutamine, glycine, taurine), and sulfur metabolites (such as from cruciferous vegetables). We can get these nutrients from our diet directly, including from herbs, as well as from supplementation.

Supporting Elimination

Did you know that you are considered constipated if you are not having a daily bowel movement?

Yep, true story. Moreover, you do not want to be detoxing if you can't eliminate properly, otherwise toxins will just recirculate in your body. Ensuring that you have proper elimination is the first step in a good detoxification process.

Diet and hydration are your first lines of defense to keep things moving through you. Adequate fiber, prebiotics/probiotics, and hydration can all support healthy gut function, optimizing digestion, assimilation, and elimination. See Chapter 12 for more details on a fertility-friendly diet.

PRECONCEPTION TIP

With hydration, aim for half of your body weight in ounces each day as a starting point (i.e., 75 ounces if you weigh 150 pounds). You may need to add more water and/or electrolytes if you are highly physically active or live in a warmer climate. Assess the color of your urine to determine if you're on the right track. You're aiming for light/ pale yellow.

Supporting Sweating, Circulation, and Lymphatic Drainage
Think of it this way: movement keeps things moving. We will cover this more in Chapter 14. Until then, it's important to know that both exercise and movement enhance detoxification. Regular movement practices support detoxification primarily through two of the major detox organs: skin (sweating) and lungs (breathing). Sweating helps to eliminate toxins from the body through your largest detox organ, your skin. Deep breathing helps dispel stale air from the lungs and replaces it with fresh oxygen, which supports detoxification processes. Movement also increases circulation. Certain exercises, like jumping rope, can also stimulate your lymphatic system, which supports the expulsion of waste products from your body.

PRECONCEPTION TIP

Here are a few extra-credit lifestyle practices if you want to go deeper.

- **Sauna**: If it's accessible to you, incorporating a twenty-minute sauna session a few times a week is a great way to improve circulation and support detoxification. Perspiration and respiration are natural ways our bodies expel the metabolic waste produced inside us, and saunas can help increase both of these processes. This helps our bodies to excrete toxic substances and heavy metals.

- **Enemas and colon hydrotherapy**: If you have a history of constipation or anticipate that you have a higher toxin load, then you may consider enemas/colon hydrotherapy. An enema is done in the comfort of your own home. Please make sure to use a clean kit and filtered water. Colon hydrotherapy is similar in concept to an enema, but it's conducted by a trained hydrotherapist. Make sure to look at reviews when selecting a practitioner.

- **Hot/cold contrast showers**: There are lots of different ways to do this, but two good starting options are to take a two- to five-minute cold shower or alternate twenty seconds of cold water followed by ten seconds of hot water for four to ten rounds, working your way up to about two to five minutes.

- **Skin brushing**: This can be done immediately prior to showering each day. Start at your feet and move upward. Begin brushing in long, sweeping motions toward your heart (always brush toward your heart). Brush each area several times. It should feel a bit prickly but invigorating.

> • **Abdominal massage:** For females specifically, abdominal massage (either self-administered or administered by a practitioner) and castor oil packs can be great tools to reduce stagnation and increase uterine blood flow.

Keep in mind: you don't have to do all of these things. The foundational practices are hydration, diet, supplementation, and movement. After that, you can pick the techniques that are most interesting and doable for you and your lifestyle.

ELECTROMAGNETIC FREQUENCY EXPOSURE

A conversation on optimizing your environment would not be complete without discussing EMFs (or electromagnetic frequencies). EMFs are produced by electrically charged objects like your phone, laptop, and Wi-Fi router. This is a whole topic unto itself, so I will keep this section brief. There are three things that you need to know:

1. EMFs Are Everywhere and Only Increasing in Prevalence

Electronic devices enable incredible connectivity and efficiency. However, the proliferation in the number of devices with EMFs and the frequency with which we use these devices has dramatically increased our exposure to EMF radiation in the past few decades. Common sources of EMFs include:

- Computers
- Cell phones
- Cell towers
- Wi-Fi routers
- Wi-Fi-enabled appliances
- Bluetooth-enabled devices

2. EMFs Have Been Shown to Impact Fertility

EMFs increase oxidative stress in your body, which can impair both egg and sperm health. In particular, studies have shown that EMFs negatively affect sperm quality across various dimensions, including sperm count, motility, and morphology.[29]

Studies have found that radio frequency electromagnetic radiation emitted from cell phones may impact sperm concentration.[30] The same may be true of wireless internet use and sperm count.[31] More research is clearly needed here. In the meantime, let's just be practical—get the phone out of your pocket and the laptop off your lap as much as possible.

3. You Have to Take Proactive Action to Reduce Your EMF Exposure

At the time of this writing, we are transitioning from 4G to 5G. The number of Wi-Fi-enabled devices continues to increase. Wi-Fi connectivity is unlikely to reverse. As with most of the items in this chapter, you are going to have to take your health into your own hands. A great place to start is minimizing EMF exposures in your own home—both the sources of exposure and frequency of exposure. See

9monthsisnotenough.com/bookresources for more resources on EMFs.

That was a lot of information! I know that thinking about detoxing your life can feel overwhelming, and I honor that. I've been there myself. You may feel as though you've already made great strides in this area. Or you may feel like you have a lot of work to do to detoxify your life. Take comfort in the fact that your body is incredibly resilient. To demonstrate just how resilient, one interventional study showed that switching to an organic diet lowered pesticide metabolites in urine by 60–95 percent, depending on the compound, after only six days.[32]

Once you start to make these changes, your body responds. Blood levels, in particular, respond quickly to dietary and lifestyle changes. It usually takes longer to clear out cell, bone and fat stores, but that's exactly why we are starting early and giving your body plenty of time before baby!

It's never too early to reduce toxin exposures. Depending on the compound, it can take a while to excrete from the body, and some compounds require an active rather than passive process (e.g., heavy metals like mercury, mold). For higher detox loads or for persistent compounds, it is best addressed in partnership with a skilled practitioner who has experience working with safe detoxification protocols for these compounds.

Take your time and refer to the resources at *9monthsisnotenough.com/bookresources* for additional support. You've got this!

CHAPTER SUMMARY

- Our bodies naturally detoxify themselves, but they cannot keep up with the volume and pace of new chemicals bombarding us on a daily basis.

- Current environmental toxin regulations are entirely too lax. If you want to optimize health and fertility, it is imperative to take personal responsibility for your exposures until regulations catch up.

- Major sources of toxic exposures include air, water, food, personal care products, and home care products. EMFs are also becoming more prevalent.

- The two ways to support detoxification are to decrease toxic exposures and increase detox capacity.

- It is not recommended to detox during pregnancy. Start your detox regimen well in advance of trying to conceive.

- If you feel you have significant exposures and would like to do a more concerted detoxification regimen, please work with a certified healthcare practitioner, and do it far in advance of conceiving.

THE FERTILE ZONE
Rightsize Your Body Composition for Conception and Pregnancy

To understand whether your weight is impacting your health, we can look at several different markers.

If you are overweight or obese, your metabolic status and hormone status in particular are helpful benchmarks.

- Metabolic Status
  - Blood Sugar Management (Glucose, Hemoglobin A1c, Insulin)
  - Cholesterol Metabolism (Lipid Panel)
  - Inflammatory Markers (hs-CRP)
- Hormone Status
  - Reproductive Hormones (DHEA-Sulfate, Estradiol, Free/Total Testosterone, FSH, LH, Sex Hormone Binding Globulin[1])

- Stress Hormones (Cortisol)
- Thyroid Function (TSH, Free/Total T3, Free/Total T4)
- Nutrient Status (Omega-3 and Omega-6 Fatty Acids, Vitamin D)

If you are underweight, we want to look at your nutrient status and hormone status in particular, as well as thyroid function, since that can be depleted with low nutrient status:

- Nutrient Status (Folate, Vitamin B12, Vitamin D)
- Hormone Status (DHEA Sulfate, Estradiol, Free/Total Testosterone, LH, FSH, and Cortisol)
- Thyroid Function (TSH, Free/Total T3, Free/ Total T4)

In addition to body fat and waist-to-hip ratio, we can use these lab markers to determine if your weight is indicative of other problems. All these markers will give a much better picture of your underlying health than weight alone ever could.

Please note: In this chapter, I am going to use the clinical classifications for "underweight" (body mass index, or BMI < 18.5), "overweight" (BMI of 25–29.9), and "obese" (BMI > 30).

$$BMI = (\text{weight in pounds} \times 703)/(\text{height in inches})^2$$

A few thoughts on this: First, I am not a huge fan of BMI measurements. They are overly simplified and are only one measure of a person's "health status." For body composition, I prefer body fat measurements. That being said, most of the clinical studies on this topic have been done with BMI, so we have to work with the data we have.

Second, as someone who has run hundreds of lab tests on clients, I recognize that weight tends to be a proxy for overall health status. This is not always the case, and I fully acknowledge that. However, in the absence of clinical data, weight status is one of the leading metrics we have to use right now. I hope that changes in the future, but until then, let's use the information we have to make as informed decisions as possible.

Last, and perhaps most important, having worked as a nutritionist with an advanced certification in eating psychology, I recognize how complex of a topic weight and associated body image can be. I want to approach this topic with deep compassion. I also want to give you the facts, as we understand them, from a clinical lens. Please take from this chapter what best serves you. If you would like more support on this topic, please see 9monthsisnotenough.com/bookresources.

Weight matters in two main ways: the amount of fat tissue itself has implications on fertility and pregnancy, and weight can act as a proxy for health status. The high-level takeaway is that being overweight/obese *or* being underweight can impair fertility, but for different reasons. In fact, according to the American Society for Reproductive Medicine (ASRM), having either too low or too high of a body weight was shown to contribute to 12 percent of infertility cases.[2]

HOW BEING OVERWEIGHT/
OBESE AFFECTS FERTILITY

Did you know that fat is not inert tissue? It is hormonally active tissue. Essentially, the more body fat you have, the more estrogen your body produces.[3] Because of this, excess body fat can predispose you to a higher estrogenic state, which can interfere with ovulation. If you are overweight, you may also have issues with blood sugar management or nutrient deficiencies. Since your hormonal system is so delicate, any imbalances can impact fertility. Being overweight can contribute to problems with getting pregnant (due to irregular ovulation or periods), staying pregnant (due to decreased egg quality and increased miscarriage risk), and having a healthy pregnancy (due to complications).

Maternal obesity increases health risks for both mother and baby during pregnancy as well. For the baby, there is an increased risk of stillbirth, congenital abnormalities, macrosomia, and preterm birth. For the mother, there is an increased risk of preeclampsia and gestational diabetes, as well as labor and delivery complications, including Cesarean delivery.[4] Given the health complications associated with obesity (likely due to the correlation between obesity and metabolic syndrome), it is probably not surprising to know that those complications can also affect a potential pregnancy.

HOW BEING UNDERWEIGHT AFFECTS FERTILITY

Being underweight can contribute to problems with ovulation and irregular menstrual periods. Having too low body fat indicates to your body that you are "starving," and your body then diverts resources from making your sex hormones to making stress hormones. This means you don't have the raw materials to make adequate sex hormones, which can impact ovulation.

Further, in early pregnancy, the embryo undergoes incredibly rapid growth that depends on maternal nutrient stores, but you can't give what you don't have. *In effect, the baby's development in the first one to two months of pregnancy is dependent on what the mother ate in the two to three months prior to pregnancy.* If the maternal nutrient stores are insufficient at conception, the placenta will likely never have a chance to develop properly. If the placenta is unable to develop properly, the fetus will not receive optimal nourishment, *regardless of the mother's nutrient intake later in pregnancy.* This is one of the reasons you see risks such as growth retardation and low birthweight in underweight mothers. It's important to note that this can and often does happen in normal weight or overweight women with nutrient-poor diets or inadequate supplementation. In effect, they are not getting the nutrition they need from the food that they eat, so their bodies are overfed with "empty" calories but starving for real nutrients.

Being underweight during pregnancy has increased risks too. For the baby, there is an increased risk of preterm birth, intrauterine growth retardation, and low birthweight.[5] Low birthweight babies have higher risks for infant mortality, sight and hearing problems, and learning difficulties. For the mother, there is an increased risk of anemia and osteoporosis.

IMPLICATIONS OF BEING
EITHER OVERWEIGHT OR
UNDERWEIGHT ON YOUR BABY

There are two main implications: birth size and fetal development.

On Birth Size

In both cases, the mother's weight has an impact on the baby's birth size. *Why do we care about birth size?* Because size at birth is related to the risk of developing disease later in life. Both large for gestational age (LGA), which is associated with overweight/obese women, and small for gestational age (SGA), which is associated with underweight women, are associated with potential health complications for the child.[6]

On Fetal Development

When I was getting my master's in nutrition, I came across a passage that radically changed my view of pregnancy. From *Nutrition Through the Life Cycle* by Judith Brown:

> The fetus is not a "parasite"—the fetus cannot take whatever nutrients it needs from the mother's body at the mother's expense. When maternal nutrient intakes fall below optimum levels…fetal growth and development are compromised more than maternal health. In general, nutrients will first be used to support maternal nutrient needs for her health and physiological changes, and next for placental development, before they become

available at optimal levels to the fetus...the fetus is generally harmed more by poor maternal nutritional status than the mother.[7]

Really? This means that your body will preferentially take care of your nutrient needs over your baby's nutrient needs. Though this seems to go against the core maternal instinct to protect your baby at all costs, it makes intuitive sense as a survival instinct. Your body will always preserve your well-being above all else. It's just like in airplanes when they tell you to put your oxygen mask on first in case of emergency. That's exactly what your body does with nutrients—it puts your nutrients "on first" so that you are healthy and capable enough to take care of others. In most cases, a baby can't survive and thrive if its mama can't survive and thrive.

Being underweight *or* overweight may indicate that you have nutrient deficiencies.

What are the implications of this?

- If you have nutrient deficiencies going into pregnancy, your body will try to rectify those nutrient deficiencies in your body first. In other words, if you have low vitamin D and begin taking a vitamin D supplement, your body will use that to replenish your body's vitamin D stores rather than passing most of it on to the baby.

- If you are underweight, your body will put on weight at the expense of the baby's growth.

- If you don't nourish yourself properly during pregnancy (both in quantity and quality of food), your baby will suffer the consequences more profoundly than you do.

As you can see, both overweight/obese and underweight women carry an increased risk for adverse pregnancy outcomes, but for different reasons.

If you are overweight or obese, *it is important to address your weight and nutrient status prior to getting pregnant* since losing weight during pregnancy is not advised. Appropriate weight loss and nutritional intake before pregnancy reduces many of the risks listed above considerably.

If you are underweight (or undernourished based on your lab results), *it is important to address your weight and nutrient status prior to getting pregnant* since your body will be preferentially nourished over your baby's body.

In both cases, you want to make these adjustments *before* you get pregnant.

One last note: if you have a tendency toward both under-eating and overexercising (which many of my clients did when they first came to see me), then that approach is likely not compatible with optimal fertility. This tendency amplifies the likelihood of nutrient deficiencies and dysregulated hormones. It may have worked well for you in previous chapters of life, but it may need to be tweaked to set you up for a successful conception and pregnancy if that's what you now desire.

IMPLICATIONS OF WEIGHT
ON SPERM QUALITY

Weight is also a factor for male reproductive partners. One recent meta-analysis confirmed that there is a direct correlation between obesity and sperm count. Specifically, sperm count falls 2.4 percent for every five-unit increase in BMI.[8] Based on this, we can anticipate that increased body mass index has a negative effect on sperm quality. We know that sperm quality directly affects fertility and time to pregnancy. In addition, diabetes, which is often present alongside an elevated BMI, can also impact sperm health. However, it is also important to note that both morbid obesity and being underweight have a negative effect on sperm quality.[9] As is often the case with health, the middle road tends to be the most effective and sustainable. Normal body weight is the best foundation for fertility.

WHY DO I NEED TO ADDRESS MY
WEIGHT BEFORE PREGNANCY?

For females, trying to lose weight during pregnancy causes two main problems. First, if you try to limit your food intake to control your weight, your body will preferentially "feed" your body over your baby's body. If there isn't enough nutrition to go around, your body will use the nutrition that is available for your needs first. We know this because there have been several studies that have shown newborns with vitamin or mineral deficiencies while their mothers don't present with these same vitamin or mineral deficiencies.

Therefore, if you restrict calories during pregnancy, your baby is likely not to have sufficient nutrition to grow and will likely not develop normally. Second, many toxins are stored in our fat tissue. When we lose weight, these toxins (such as persistent organic pollutants) are liberated into our bloodstream.[10] We don't want this to be happening while we are pregnant.

For males, the only biological contribution you are making to the baby is at conception, so this is your one shot (literally) to contribute the best raw materials you possibly can.

Now that we've talked about why it's important to optimize body composition, let's talk about how to figure out the right range for you.

WHAT CAN YOU DO TO OPTIMIZE BODY COMPOSITION FOR FERTILITY?

The optimal BMI range for pregnancy is aligned with the "normal" BMI range for women from 18.5–24.9. As discussed above, body fat is an even better indicator of optimal body composition. I suggest aiming for the "fertile zone" to optimize chances of conceiving. It will be slightly different for everyone, but around 16–26 percent body fat is a decent guideline for females and 6–17 percent for males, depending on age, body type, and other health parameters. In partnership with your doctor, I recommend that you look at the lab markers mentioned earlier in the chapter to determine your current status and come up with a plan to achieve the optimal body fat range for your body.

THE FERTILE ZONE

PRECONCEPTION TIP

To measure body fat at home, you can use either skinfold calipers or a handheld bioelectrical imped-ance device (BIA), which sends a weak electric current through the body to calculate impedance (resistance). Muscle tissue has lower impedance than fat tissue, which is how body composition is calculated. To get the most accurate reading with a BIA, make sure to hydrate well before using.

I do not want to gloss over or oversimplify the topic of weight loss. That could be a book unto itself!

However, as a nutritionist and a personal trainer, what I will say is this:

1. Nutrition is your first line of defense.
2. When nutrition alone isn't cutting it, look at lab work.
3. Exercise is fantastic for many things (see Chapter 14), but fat loss is not really one of them.

I find that there are usually two main elements to fat loss: physiological and psychological/emotional. In this book, we are primarily focusing on the physiological components. Often, what I see with clients is that once they've made many of the upgrades suggested throughout this book (e.g., diet, supplementation, detoxification) and addressed any underlying chronic health conditions, weight tends to normalize to a healthy range on its own. However, with my eating psychology coach hat on, I recognize that's only one piece of the puzzle. If you would like access to more resources on the eating psychology front, see *9monthsis notenough.com/bookresources.*

CHAPTER SUMMARY

- Both being underweight and being overweight can interfere with fertility and pregnancy outcomes.

- Using lab markers can be a much more effective way to know if you need to address your weight rather than relying on BMI alone.

- If you need to address your weight, it should be done *before* conceiving.

THE FOUNDATION OF FERTILITY

Decode and Optimize Your Menstrual Cycle

STATUS CHECK

We can measure a whole host of biomarkers that can impact your reproductive health and fertility. Since your fertility is an extension of your overall health, biomarkers across all five categories will influence it. Here is a shortlist to pay particular attention to:

- Blood Status (CBC, Ferritin) can indicate if you are losing an excessive amount of iron.
- Hormone Status can help us understand what is driving your menstrual cycle and whether your endocrine system is in optimal working order for conception and pregnancy.

- Reproductive Hormones (DHEAS, Estradiol, Free/Total Testosterone, FSH, LH, Prolactin, and SHBG for females, as well as Dihydrotestosterone for males)
- Stress Hormones (Cortisol)
- Thyroid Function (TSH, Free/Total T3, Free/Total T4, Reverse T3)
- Immune Status (STI Screening) can help us understand if there are any underlying infections impacting your fertility.
- Metabolic Status can give us a window into ovulation and egg/sperm quality and help us understand how your body is processing hormones.
  - Blood Sugar Management (Glucose, Hemoglobin A1c, Insulin)
  - Liver Function (Albumin, ALT, AST)

We spend so much of life trying *not* to get pregnant. In that phase of life, getting a period each month usually brings a sigh of relief. Then one day, we flip the script. We decide that it's time to conceive, and we expect our bodies to comply. Sometimes it works. Sometimes it doesn't. This book is here to help increase the probability that it works.

Beyond being an indicator of pregnancy or not, our menstrual cycles also convey a lot of information. They are an indicator of your overall health status. According to Lara Briden, ND, the menstrual cycle has been called a "monthly report card" and the "fifth vital sign" (alongside body temperature, blood pressure, pulse/heart rate, and respiration rate). Your period is a gold mine of information if you observe it and track it.

In essence, the healthier you are, the healthier your periods are. More importantly for us, the healthier your periods are, the more fertile you are. A regular, healthy period is the foundation of fertility. For this reason, exploring and troubleshooting your period (and associated symptoms) is a critical part of your conception journey.

WHAT IS A "NORMAL" PERIOD?

Understanding how your cycle works is the first step in troubleshooting it. Normal menstrual cycle length ranges from around twenty-one to thirty-five days (for 80 percent of women). No, not every woman's cycle is the proverbial twenty-eight days, so you can let that go right now.

The first day of your period is the first day of your menstrual cycle. Some women experience spotting before their period; this is not counted as the first day of your cycle— it's the first day of fresh, red blood. The menstrual cycle is counted from the first day of one period to the day before the next period.

There are two main phases in a menstrual cycle: the follicular phase (before ovulation) and the luteal phase (after ovulation). The day of ovulation determines how long your cycle is. The length of the follicular phase can vary widely, usually anywhere from seven to twenty-one days. However, the length of the luteal phase is usually fourteen days (or less) because that is how long the corpus luteum can survive without a pregnancy. The corpus luteum is a progesterone-secreting structure that develops in an ovary after an egg has been discharged for ovulation; it disappears after a few days unless pregnancy occurs.

> *Please note: If your luteal phase is much shorter than fourteen days, you are likely experiencing luteal phase defect, which can prevent implantation because it doesn't give the embryo enough time to attach inside the uterus.*

Here are the key characteristics of a regular (or normal) period and an irregular period:

	Regular period	Irregular period
Timing	• Around three- to seven-day menstruation • Cycle arrives around every twenty-one to thirty-five days • Ovulation is around twelve to fourteen days prior to menstruation	• No period, long period • Short cycles, long cycles • No ovulation
Flow	• Bright red color • Syrup-like consistency • No large clots • Moderate flow (~50mL blood)[1]	• Frequent colors besides red (e.g., deep brown, black, purple, pink)[2] • Excessively thin or thick consistency • Large clots • Light flow (< 25 mL) or heavy flow (> 80 mL)
Symptoms	• Minimal to no PMS • Minimal to no period pain	• Significant PMS • Significant period pain

FAQ: BUT WAIT! WHEN SHOULD I GO OFF HORMONAL BIRTH CONTROL?

You will want to discuss any medication changes with your doctor. If you and your doctor decide that discontinuing birth control is right for you, then you will want to use an alternative form of birth control (such as condoms or diaphragms) until you are ready to conceive.

Keep in mind that discontinuing birth control is an active process, not a passive one. In most cases, you can't just stop birth control and everything will kick-start again. You will need to take targeted actions (including supplementation) and do some troubleshooting. It usually requires more time than people anticipate, so give yourself a liberal runway.

If you have just come off hormonal birth control, your primary objective is to restore a normal, regular period each month. As a reminder from Chapter 2, birth control can mask underlying hormonal imbalances while you are on it. Even once you're off it, the effects of hormonal birth control can increase barriers to—and therefore time to—getting pregnant. It can take up to a year to restore healthy hormonal balance and a regular period after going off birth control. Given this, you want to give yourself some time to transition off birth control and ensure that your hormonal system is in good shape before trying to conceive.

According to Dr. Jolene Brighten, an expert on post-birth control syndrome:

> ..."post-birth control syndrome" is a term that refers to the collection of signs and symptoms

that arise when you stop taking the pill. These can be symptoms you were suppressing with the pill, or they can be added side effects the pill created that your body is waking up to.[3]

These symptoms include but are not limited to headaches, mood swings, depression and anxiety, acne, polycystic ovary syndrome (PCOS), hypothyroidism, amenorrhea, leaky gut, and dysregulated immune function.

Why? Dr. Brighten explains that:

...the basic mechanism of the pill is to flood your body with enough hormones that your brain stops communicating with your ovaries and you cease to ovulate. If the pill shuts down the conversation between your ovaries and your brain, then it's no surprise that once you stop taking it you may encounter some challenges reestablishing the connection—not to mention the strain it has created on your adrenal, thyroid, gut, and liver. And that can have some long-term effects if you've taken the pill for a substantial amount of time.[4]

This is the case with most of the clients I've worked with who have been on the pill for years.

Because it can take time to clear out the effects of hormonal birth control, I suggest giving yourself plenty of time—ideally at least six to nine months.

If you're just now deciding to come off hormonal birth control, this entire pre-pregnancy checklist is designed to help you work through many of the things that can remedy post-birth control syndrome, including reducing your toxic load, supporting your liver function, modulating stress, healing your gut, restoring your hormone levels, repleting nutrients, and so on. You are already well on your way. Just give yourself enough time and grace as you work through the process of reigniting your brain–ovarian communication mechanism.

If you have been off hormonal birth control for some time (or were never on it), your primary objective is to make sure that you are having a seamless (read: pain-free and mostly symptom-free) period each month.

In both cases, you want to start to track and monitor ovulation. In the next section, we will discuss how to figure out if you are ovulating.

AM I OVULATING?

Generally, females ovulate once per cycle. Ovulation appears to occur randomly from either the left or right ovary. Occasionally, eggs are ovulated from both ovaries (which is how fraternal twins happen). If you ovulate more than once, it will likely occur within twenty-four hours.

Despite what you may have heard, you can get your period without ovulating. A period is *not* a definite sign that ovulation has occurred. Just because you had your period does *not* necessarily mean that you ovulated.

Most females ovulate between days six and twenty (based on average cycle length of twenty-one to thirty-five days). Luteinizing hormone (LH) surges around twenty-four to thirty-six hours before ovulation. To figure out when you ovulate, it is more accurate to count back around fifteen days from your current period than forward fourteen days from your last period (again, because the luteal phase is fairly constant while the follicular phase can vary widely). It can take a while to get the hang of this, so it's helpful to track for several months.

There are several natural indicators and technological indicators you can use to gauge ovulation.

Natural Indicators

- **Cervical mucus**: Raw egg white consistency ("fertile mucus")
- **Temperature**: Basal body temperature (BBT) rises 0.5–1.0 degrees Fahrenheit after ovulation (*Note:* if you choose to track BBT, you will need a special thermometer or device designed specifically for this purpose)
- **Cervix position**: SHOW (soft, high, open, wet)

Other potential, but not definitive, signs of ovulation include increased sexual desire, breast tenderness, slight spotting, ovulation twinges, and heightened senses.

Technological Indicators

- **Ovulation predictor kit (OPK)**: Measures surge in LH
- **Saliva ferning microscope**: Observes "ferning" of saliva during LH surge
- **Fertility monitor**: Measures cycle length (including luteal phase length), temperature changes, and ovulation

It is up to you how you would like to monitor ovulation; however, I would encourage you to pick a method of tracking at least initially to get a sense for when you ovulate each month. You can choose which natural or technological indicators you'd like to monitor as part of this process.

PREDICTING AND
CONFIRMING OVULATION

All the measures that I just listed are leading indicators of ovulation, meaning they precede ovulation. Historically, this has been the only tool available to assess ovulation. There are new tools on the market that allow us to measure progesterone, which is produced *after* ovulation.

A quick primer on progesterone: after ovulation, the follicle from which the egg was released (the corpus luteum) starts producing progesterone. Progesterone plays many roles, but it is particularly important for sustaining a pregnancy because it helps to create the optimal uterine environment in which an embryo can thrive.

If LH predicts ovulation, progesterone confirms it happened. In many women, LH strips have been a frustratingly inaccurate predictor of ovulation because many women don't experience a clear LH surge or experience multiple LH surges.

For this reason, I recommend my clients look at both LH and progesterone if they want to understand what is going on with their cycle. You can do this with either LH and progesterone strips or fertility monitors that measure both levels. You don't need to be obsessive about it, and you don't need

> to do it for many cycles in order to figure out what's going on. This is just another tool in your toolkit to give you more information about what's going on in your body.

I can't end this section without a note on ovulation tracking apps. There are currently over two hundred ovulation trackers in the market, but the average accuracy rate hovers around 20 percent.[5] I am all for tracking and tabulating, but there just isn't good evidence to support the use of these apps. In many cases, they are extrapolating your ovulation date from the start or end date of your period, not personalizing it to your unique follicular phase, which, as we discussed, can vary widely. You can use them as a general guide, but I would not recommend relying too heavily on them for your fertility planning purposes.

WHAT CAN INTERFERE WITH REGULAR PERIODS AND OVULATION?

You've tested your ovulation, and you've found out that you're not ovulating, either at all or regularly. What next? First, breathe. This is very common and addressable in the vast majority of cases.

What might be going on? Hormones are an intimate and delicate cascade. What affects one hormone can affect the others. When your body senses lack of safety (adrenaline) or malnutrition (cortisol), it makes the decision *not* to ovulate because it believes you're not in a safe environment to bring a baby into the world.

If you want to get pregnant, you need to ovulate. It's not the only piece of the puzzle, but it's the centerpiece. Regular ovulation is foundational for fertility. Unfortunately, our modern lifestyle can be a real buzzkill when it comes to ovulation. If your body is meaningfully out of balance, it will shut down ovulation. Luckily, you're here to learn how to reverse engineer your lifestyle to be ovulation friendly.

The most common obstacles to ovulation are:

- Environmental toxins, especially endocrine disruptors and certain medications
- Suboptimal diet (leading to nutrient deficiencies, blood sugar imbalance/insulin resistance, inflammation, insufficient caloric intake)
- Stress (both psychological such as job anxiety and physiological such as underlying viruses or infections, overexercising, or restricting calories)
- Inflammation and underlying health conditions, especially immune system dysfunction and thyroid dysfunction

Ovulation is a divine but delicate process. Everything needs to go just right in order for that egg to release every month. One of the first steps in your preconception journey should be to make sure that you're ovulating regularly (and paradoxically, you want to do this without stressing yourself out too much about whether and when you're ovulating!).

HOW CAN I RESTORE OVULATION?

The pre-pregnancy checklist is designed to support optimal hormonal balance and regular ovulation. In Chapter 9, you reduced your toxin load through active detoxification. In Chapter 12, you addressed your nutrient deficiencies and blood sugar balance through your diet. In this chapter, you will be observing and tracking your menstrual cycle. Step-by-step, I am walking you through the process to restore a natural menstrual cycle and ovulation, if that hasn't been the case for you so far. I am here to guide you through the process. At the same time, I want to empower you to be your own health detective.

Your body wants to ovulate. Your body is designed to ovulate. Your body also wants to keep you and your future baby safe and sound. If you haven't been ovulating regularly (based on the natural or technological indicators discussed above), get curious. First, reflect: *What could be throwing my system off? Where are things out of balance in my life right now? What's making my body think that I'm living in an unsafe or unstable environment?* Sometimes, you will know instinctively where things went awry. It may be intense job stress or your overbearing mother-in-law. It may be heavy metal toxicity from your personal care products or your daily tuna salad (yes, that's possible!). It may be blood sugar dysregulation from too many coffee-and-muffin breakfasts.

Second, recognize that your body is trying to protect you, not sabotage you. Your body is incredibly wise; even if you don't always understand her, try to trust her. Finally, have faith that once you remove the roadblock(s), your body will restore its natural function and begin ovulating again.

Not ovulating occasionally when life gets bonkers is totally normal, but not ovulating regularly is a sign of dysfunction and will need to be addressed if you want to get pregnant. When ovulation isn't working the way it should, it's your body's way of telling you that things are out of sorts. Rather than pushing and shoving ovulation back into "working order" (e.g., with drugs or procedures), it is most effective to figure out where the roadblock is and remove that. Most of the time, your body will heal itself if it's just given the chance. Sometimes drugs and procedures are necessary, but that should ideally be a last resort rather than a first exploration.

PERIOD SYMPTOMS ARE COMMON, BUT THEY ARE NOT NORMAL

Irregular ovulation is one sign of a dysregulated menstrual cycle and is often accompanied by other period symptoms. Period symptoms usually indicate a hormonal imbalance, which can lead to ovulation challenges. If you haven't yet started monitoring ovulation and you have an irregular period or strong PMS symptoms, that can suggest issues with regular ovulation. It's important to dig into what's causing your PMS so you know how to optimize your period and, by extension, your ovulation.

Despite the fact that PMS is common, it is not normal (i.e., the way your body was designed to operate). As I outlined above, a normal period is relatively seamless and pain free. If you have lots of period symptoms, that's an indicator of an underlying hormonal imbalance.

In the table below, I highlight some of the most common symptoms of PMS and what might be causing them:

If you experience...	It's likely driven by...
Acne	High androgens (e.g., testosterone)
Bloating	High estrogen, low progesterone
Brain fog/memory issues	Estrogen imbalance (either too low or too high)
Breast tenderness	High estrogen, low progesterone
Brown spotting (prior to or between periods)	Low progesterone
Cramps	Excess prostaglandins
Dark red/black clots	High estrogen, sluggish blood flow
Depression/low mood	Estrogen imbalance (either too low or too high)
Heavy periods	High estrogen, low progesterone
Irregular cycles	Low progesterone and estrogen or high estrogen
Irritability	High estrogen
Light periods	Low estrogen
Long cycles	Excess androgens
Migraines	High estrogen, low progesterone
Short cycles	Low progesterone, sluggish thyroid
Vaginal dryness/lack of lubrication	Low estrogen and androgens

Period symptoms are one indicator of what may be going on, and you can use lab work to confirm your hypotheses.

Any of these dysregulated hormonal states can make it harder to become pregnant and would ideally be corrected before you start trying to conceive.

How to Combat the Most Common Causes of PMS

Now that you've learned about what might be causing your PMS symptoms, here is a quick "cheat sheet" on how to address these symptoms holistically.

Please note: Consult with your doctor before starting any new supplementation. These herbs and supplements may not be appropriate for use during pregnancy or breastfeeding and may have interactions with other drugs or supplements (e.g., anticoagulants). Most herbs are not recommended while trying to conceive or during pregnancy.

If You Have Too Much Estrogen and/or Androgens
Optimize Your Diet

- Balance your blood sugar.
- Reach for grass-fed, antibiotic/hormone-free animal and dairy products that are not laden with hormones like many traditional animal products.
- Incorporate foods that help detoxify estrogen and excrete it from the body (e.g., cruciferous vegetables, flaxseeds, chia seeds, fiber-rich vegetables).
- Moderate intake of alcohol and caffeine, which can tax your liver and impair its ability to clear excess hormones.
- Drink plenty of water to make sure that you are flushing things out.

Adjust Your Lifestyle

- Modify your body composition since fat cells produce estrogen, which reinforces the problem.
- Moderate your stress levels.
- Get rid of any xenoestrogens (hormone disruptors that have estrogen-like effects) that are hiding in your personal care or home care products.
- Increase your detoxification capacity (e.g., exercise regularly, get your sweat on, have regular bowel movements).
- Mind your gut microbiome since you will reabsorb estrogen if your bacteria are imbalanced.

Consider Supplementation

- DIM (diindolylmethane) which balances estrogen metabolism
- Calcium-D-glucarate which supports detoxification of toxins (including excess hormones)
- Desiccated liver and other liver-support herbs (e.g., milk thistle, dandelion root)

If You Have Too Little Progesterone and/or Estrogen
Optimize Your Diet

- Eat adequate protein, which gives your body the raw materials it needs to make hormones.
- Include healthy sources of animal fat (e.g., grass-fed butter) in your diet, which converts into cholesterol and is the foundation of all sex hormones.
- Ensure your diet is rich in nutrients that are building blocks of your sex hormones, including vitamin B6, vitamin E, zinc, and magnesium.

Adjust Your Lifestyle

- Moderate your stress levels, which can divert resources away from making sex hormones.
- Avoid overexercising, which increases cortisol.
- Avoid extreme dieting, which increases cortisol.

Consider Supplementation

- Adrenal support supplements (e.g., ashwagandha, rhodiola, holy basil)
- Thyroid support supplements
- Progesterone only: Vitex/chaste tree berry
- Estrogen only: Dong quai (please use caution if you have a family history of estrogen-sensitive cancers)

If You Have Sluggish Blood Flow
Optimize Your Diet

- Reduce inflammatory foods in your diet (e.g., vegetable oils, processed fats, factory-farmed animal products).

Adjust Your Lifestyle

- Try Mayan abdominal massage, which helps release physical blockages and restore blood flow.
- Visit an acupuncturist, who can help improve circulation to the reproductive organs.
- Get moving regularly to avoid stagnation of blood flow, especially around the reproductive organs.

Consider Supplementation

- Fish oil, which helps increase circulation

If You Have Excess Prostaglandins
Optimize Your Diet

- Moderate your intake of linoleic and arachidonic acids (e.g., corn, soy, vegetable oils), or omega-6 fats, which are precursors to prostaglandins.
- Eat adequate amounts of omega-3 fats (e.g., salmon, walnuts, chia seeds, flaxseeds).
- Include foods rich in vitamin E (e.g., sunflower seeds, almonds, hazelnuts, spinach, broccoli) for its antioxidant properties.
- Incorporate citrus fruits, which contain hesperidin, a compound that suppresses prostaglandin production.
- Minimize alcohol and caffeine intake.

Adjust Your Lifestyle

- Incorporate gentle movement (e.g., walking, yoga) into your daily routine.

Consider Supplementation

- Fish oil, which has anti-inflammatory properties
- Magnesium, which may play a role in reducing prostaglandin production
- Herbs such as white willow and feverfew

The goal for *optimal readiness* is a regular menstrual cycle with regular ovulation and a relatively seamless period. Your period comes every twenty-one to thirty-five days and lasts for two to seven days. You experience minimal PMS or period pain. You have confirmed ovulation each month.

CHAPTER SUMMARY

- Your period is a "monthly report card" of what's going on with your body.

- A regular, healthy period is the foundation of fertility.

- Just because you had a period does not mean that you ovulated. If you want to track ovulation, it is best to look at both LH to predict ovulation and progesterone to confirm ovulation.

- Period symptoms are common, but they are not normal.

- Coming off hormonal birth control is an active, not a passive, process.

(12)

EAT AS IF YOU'RE ALREADY PREGNANT

Adopt a Fertility-Friendly Diet

STATUS CHECK

To better understand how your diet is serving you, we can look at two things: inputs and outputs. You can track nutrients in the foods you eat to understand the macronutrient ratios and vitamin and mineral levels you reach daily (refer to *9months isnotenough.com/bookresources* for suggested trackers). In addition, we can measure outputs (such as weight/body fat/waist to hip ratio (WHR), as discussed in the last chapter), as well as lab markers. As you will see in this chapter, the food you eat affects much more than just your nutrient status. It can impact every single area of your health.

The markers that we want to pay particular attention to include:

- Blood Status (CBC, Ferritin)
- Hormone Status
  - Reproductive Hormones (DHEAS,
    Estradiol, Free/Total Testosterone, SHBG)
  - Stress Hormones (Cortisol)
- Immune Status (ANA)
- Metabolic Status
  - Blood Sugar Management (Glucose,
    Hemoglobin A1c, Insulin)
  - Cholesterol Metabolism (Lipid Panel)
- Nutrient Status (Folate, Omega-3/Omega-6
  Index, Vitamin B12, Vitamin D)

These biomarkers show us whether your body is appropriately digesting and assimilating nutrients from the foods you eat, whether your diet is adequate enough to support hormone production and immune function, whether your body is effectively breaking down food into blood sugar and processing it properly, and whether you're getting enough essential nutrients for optimal fertility.

I'm not going to tell you what to eat or not to eat. Even though I'm a nutritionist and people expect that from me, I don't believe in giving people more "rules" around food. However, I will share the data as I understand it and the working theory that I've arrived at and allow you to come to your own conclusions about what's right for you and your body.

If you're happy with your health and fertility, I'm happy too. If you're not, maybe it's time to consider another viewpoint of what's healthy for you to eat right now in the context of your fertility goals.

INTRODUCTION TO A
FERTILITY-FRIENDLY DIET

There is so much dietary information out there (much of it conflicting) that it can be incredibly difficult to figure out what to follow. On top of that, pregnancy is the most nutrient-intensive time in a female's entire life, so it is even more imperative to make quality nutrition a priority before, during, and immediately following pregnancy. Unfortunately, it's not as simple as following Paleo, low-carb/keto, or vegan/vegetarian diets. In fact, many of these popular diets are not well suited for fertility since they do not have adequate nutritional profiles to support optimal hormonal balance. Given that, I have designed a fertility-specific diet that combines my clinical experience and the latest scientific literature into a single, comprehensive diet that sets the stage for a healthy conception and pregnancy and, ultimately, a healthy baby.

At the most basic level, the building blocks for hormones are found in the foods we eat. High-quality food is your #1 tool for supporting your fertility. Despite the fact that we will be supplementing your diet with targeted nutrients, you cannot out-supplement a poor diet. Your diet is plan A, plan B, and plan C for supporting your fertility. Supplementation is a backup plan and an added insurance policy given the intense nutrient needs required during pregnancy. A fertility diet is a core foundation of preconception preparation. It's designed to support hormonal balance, blood sugar regulation, and liver detoxification and to minimize inflammation.

WHY DOES DIET MATTER?

Studies show that "the nutritional status of both women and men before conception has profound implications for the growth, development, and long-term health of their offspring."[1]

Essentially, nutrition provides three functions: *infrastructure*, providing the scaffolding for your cell membranes (including eggs and sperm); *information*, communicating to your body that it's safe to reproduce; and *intermediaries*, or cofactors, that help your body execute important metabolic functions (like digesting food, building tissue, and creating immune cells). Because of this, females on healthy diets have been shown to have better pregnancy outcomes than those on poor diets.

Your diet provides the raw materials needed to make your hormones, which control ovulation and menstrual cycles in females and sperm development in males. Your diet can also regulate your hormones or dysregulate your hormones based on how you manage your blood sugar. The composition of your diet can send signals to your body as to whether it is a safe and abundant environment in which to conceive; eating too much or eating too little are both detrimental. Food quality also affects egg and sperm quality.

Once you conceive, the food you eat literally builds the cells in your body and the cells in your baby's body. Crappy food = crappy cells. The structure of a cell impacts its function; poor-quality raw materials lead to poor-quality cell structure, which leads to poorly functioning cells. Think of a house that's made from high-quality steel or bricks versus a house that's composed of old, rotting wood. What you eat can either be a building block or an impediment to your baby's growth.

The food we eat becomes the raw materials for our bodily tissues. The major macronutrients (fat, protein, and carbohydrates) you take in through your diet become the cells in your body. Dietary fats are converted into cell membranes, steroid hormones, myelin (the material around our nerve cells), padding, and insulation for your internal organs, as well as energy stores. Protein is converted into bones, muscles, skin, blood, hormones, enzymes, and antibodies. In addition to being a fuel source, carbohydrates are building blocks for DNA and RNA (which house your genetic material), as well as being a constituent of hormones, enzymes, and vitamins. The quality of the food we eat dictates the quality of our body.

Similarly, the quality of your food dictates the quality of your baby's body. Your fat intake affects your baby's cell membranes, brain and nervous system development, and retinal tissue. Your protein intake helps build all of the cells of your baby's body, including their blood vessels, skin, hair, nails, heart, and lungs. Your carbohydrate intake can affect your baby's birthweight and propensity for fat stores. Beyond this, vitamins also play a role in creating your baby's body. The most well-known example is folate, which plays a role in ensuring the neural tube closes properly.[2] Minerals such as calcium, phosphorus, and magnesium are key components in the baby's skeletal development.[3] This doesn't even begin to explore the impact of the many phytonutrients on your baby's cellular development.

For all of these reasons, the quality and quantity of your diet is essential to a healthy conception and pregnancy. Studies have shown that dietary interventions can be as effective as assisted reproductive techniques in supporting fertility. I'll say that again because it is so profound— dietary interventions have proven to be *as effective as assisted reproductive techniques* in supporting fertility. In the Nurses' Health Study, women who followed the principles of a fertility diet alongside other health lifestyle behaviors decreased ovulatory infertility by ~70 percent.[4] Suffice it to say, food is the foundation of a fertile lifestyle.

There is no one right diet, but as Hillary Wright, Director of Nutrition Counseling at Domar Center and Boston IVF, said, "The best diet to maximize your fertility is one that sends the strongest message to your reproductive system that says 'this is a healthy body that is a good place to reproduce.'"[5] I ascribe to that theory and have created these fertility diet guidelines to communicate to your body that it is in a safe, abundant environment in which to conceive.

It's also important to keep in mind that eating for fertility is not the same thing as eating for daily life. Nim Barnes, founder of Foresight, sums it up well: "It has been found that in all types of animal life, from insect to mammal, a diet which supports normal adult life is not necessarily sufficient to support reproduction." Barnes continues, "Besides taking in extra calories for growth and energy, you need extra vitamins, minerals, essential fatty acids and amino acids."[6]

Most females I've worked with are familiar with diets as a tool for weight management. In most cases, diets are focused on *what to remove* from your daily eating plan. In this case, diets are single purpose and used to minimize perceived downside (e.g., weight gain). But what if we could also use diets to maximize upside? While it is important to understand which foods can interfere with fertility outcomes and should therefore be minimized in your diet, it's even more important to focus on *what to add* to your eating plan for optimal fertility.

WHAT IS A FERTILITY DIET?

Your fertility diet will consist of a combination of macronutrients (protein, carbohydrates, fats) and micronutrients (vitamins, minerals, phytochemicals).

The optimal macronutrient ratio for fertility and pregnancy is:

- Moderate to high fat intake
- Moderate complex carbohydrate intake
- Moderate protein intake

Moderate to High Fat Intake

Dietary fat has been maligned in the media for years. We were told that "fat would make us fat" or that "fat would clog our arteries," but the story isn't quite that simple—and it's certainly not the most nutritionally sound advice for fertility and pregnancy. Adequate levels of healthy fats are absolutely critical for maintaining a regular menstrual cycle.

It is also important to understand that all sex hormones are made from cholesterol, which is mainly found in animal products. In other words, cholesterol is a precursor in the production of estrogen, progesterone, and testosterone, all of which are needed for reproduction. Without adequate cholesterol, your body does not have the "raw materials" necessary to make sufficient sex hormones.

The most important nuance in the fat discussion, however, is that the *variety* and *quality* of fat is what really matters when it comes to overall health and reproduction. Instead of trans fats (in items like packaged snacks and fast food), which mess with hormone signaling and have been associated with infertility, opt for a balance of saturated fats (e.g., dairy and animal meat) and unsaturated fats (e.g., olive oil and avocados), both of which are needed for healthy hormone production and signaling. Finally, when it comes to quantity, aim for the Goldilocks principle: not too much, not too little, right in the middle.

Moderate Complex Carbohydrate Intake

The Goldilocks principle applies to carbohydrates as well. Too many carbohydrates can contribute to blood sugar and insulin dysregulation issues, which can ultimately interfere with ovulation. On the other hand, too few carbohydrates can signal "scarcity" and "survival" to your body, which then shuttles resources from making your sex hormones to making your stress hormones. When this happens, your body doesn't have adequate sex hormones to menstruate regularly or reproduce. Adequate "slow carbohydrate" intake (e.g., high-fiber carbs like vegetables and whole grains) is necessary to signal to your body that it's safe and stable enough to reproduce.

Moderate Protein Intake

Dietary protein is converted into structural tissues (e.g., bones, muscles, skin) as well as blood, hormones, enzymes, and antibodies. For fertility specifically, adequate protein intake is necessary to maintain hormone levels (and to eventually maintain a pregnancy). Similar to the fat discussion above, the quality of your protein sources is super important; you want to minimize exposure to growth hormones, antibiotics, and pesticides.

In summary, a "fertility-friendly" nutrition plan includes:

- Adequate high-quality sources of saturated fat (e.g., animal fats such as dairy, eggs, beef, pork, and lamb and plant fats such as coconut and cacao butter) and unsaturated fat (e.g., animal fats such as oily fish and plant fats such as avocados, olives, nuts, and seeds)
- Moderate amounts of "slow carbohydrates" (including lots of colorful, organic produce)
- Clean sources of animal protein (e.g., grass-fed, pastured, organic, wild) and plant protein

These real foods will provide your body with the necessary macronutrients (protein, carbs, and fats) and micronutrients (vitamins, minerals, and phytonutrients) to make the appropriate levels of sex hormones to sustain a regular period and a successful pregnancy.

Ideally, the goal of a fertility diet is to eat the most nutrient-dense foods that you possibly can. That being said, we also want to be realistic and have you do what you can from your starting point. This outline is meant to be a guideline, not a prescription. However, the more closely you adhere to the dietary guidelines, the faster you are likely to see results. It is completely up to you to decide the timing and trade-offs.

Without further ado, here is an overview of the foods in each category of our fertility diet:

Fertility Friends (prioritize this!)	Fertility Foes (minimize this!)
• Organic vegetables	• Sugar (in all forms)
• Herbs and spices	• Highly processed/packaged food
• Nuts and seeds	• Fast food
• Minimally processed oils	• Non-organic meat and dairy
• Organic, pastured meat and dairy	• High-mercury fish
• Low-mercury fish/seafood	• Non-organic vegetables and fruit (especially the "Dirty Dozen"[7])
• Organic fruit	• Processed vegetable fats (margarine, shortening) and vegetable oils (canola, corn, cottonseed, soybean)
• Whole grains and legumes	
• Filtered water	
• Unsweetened tea	• Too much caffeine
• Natural sweeteners	• Too much alcohol

In addition to the Fertility Friends above, we also have a list of Fertility Favorites. These are foods that are particularly nutrient dense and hormonally supportive. I have included both the recommended foods and suggested frequency:

• Organic vegetables (especially dark, leafy greens): three to five servings per day

- Organ meats (especially liver): one to two servings per week
- Bone broth: three to five servings per week
- Organic, grass-fed eggs: three to five servings per week
- Organic, grass-fed butter and ghee: two to three servings per week
- Avocado: three to five servings per week
- Low-mercury, fatty fish (anchovies, herring, mackerel, salmon, sardines, trout, whitefish): two to three servings per week
- Olive and coconut oil: daily
- Fermented foods (e.g., sauerkraut, kimchi, pickles): daily
- Slow carbs (including starchy vegetables and sprouted grains/legumes): daily
- Seeds: two to three servings per week
- Methyl donors and methylation adaptogens (e.g., beets, liver, turmeric, rosemary, green tea, cruciferous vegetables): daily

There you have it!

Now that we've covered the basics of a fertility-friendly diet, I am going to dive deeper into some specific topics that have arisen as common questions from clients over the years.

Spotlight On: Organic Food

The organic debate is a heated one. Is it really any better? Does it really make a difference? Is it worth the money?

Yes, yes, and yes. Organic food is *not* a fad. Don't just take my word for it. Let's talk numbers.

A groundbreaking meta-analysis found organic produce to be:

- ~20–70 percent higher in antioxidants than conventional produce, depending on type of antioxidant
- Four times lower in pesticides than conventional produce
- Lower in heavy metals (cadmium specifically) than conventional produce[8]

In terms of organic animal products:

- Organic milk was found to have a more desirable fatty acid composition than conventional milk, including higher omega-3 fats and conjugated linoleic acid[9]
- Both organic milk and meat contain ~50 percent more beneficial omega-3 fatty acids than conventionally produced products[10]
- Organic meat and dairy also cannot contain synthetic hormones (e.g., rBGH), which have been associated with an increased risk of breast, colon, and prostate cancers (though the research is inconclusive to date)[11]

In summary, organic produce and animal products are higher in antioxidants and omega-3 fats and lower in pesticides and heavy metals.

Why should you care? Aside from the broad health benefits of antioxidants and omega-3 fats and the potential health detriments of pesticides and heavy metals, these factors are particularly relevant for fertility and pregnancy because:

- **Antioxidants boost egg and sperm health.** Both egg and sperm quality can be improved by key antioxidants (e.g., CoQ10, vitamin E), which reduce oxidative stress.

- **Omega-3 fats support cardiovascular, immune, and neurodevelopmental health.** Omega-3s are linked to a reduction in cardiovascular disease risk as well as an improvement in neurological and immune development and function. They also support a baby's brain development during pregnancy.

- **Pesticides are linked to low sperm parameters.** One study found that "on average, men in the highest quartile of high pesticide residue fruits and vegetables had 49% lower total sperm count, 32% fewer morphologically normal sperm and 29% lower ejaculate volume than men in the lowest quartile of intake."[12] In addition, several studies have found elevated rates of infertility among farm workers exposed to high amounts of pesticides.[13]

- **Excess heavy metal levels are linked to fertility challenges.** High heavy metal levels have been shown to impair fertility in women and men.[14]

I hope it's clear that the benefits of organic food are substantial.

Beyond that, it's important to recognize that the "organic" distinction is a relatively new one. A few hundred years ago, *everything* was organic. Our ancestors were all eating organic produce and animal products because that's all there was. Their food was unadulterated by pesticides, antibiotics, hormones, and genetic modification. Food was just food. No distinctions, delineations, or labels.

In fact, there is nothing "conventional" about conventional produce and animal products. We didn't evolve eating pesticides, antibiotics, hormones, and genetically modified organisms (GMOs). These are all relatively new to our system, and we aren't assimilating them so well.

I'd invite you to reframe this discussion about organic. It's not really a question of whether organic is better for our bodies or not. It's a question of public policy (how our agricultural standards and subsidies will evolve) and a question of personal choice (how you choose to spend your agricultural dollars).

Until we have more widespread policy changes, it's up to you to decide how much of a priority organic food will be in your spending budget. This will be different for everyone and will depend on several variables, including access to organic food, price constraints, and health status. It's not about being 100 percent organic 100 percent of the time, but it is about being an informed consumer and making proactive choices with the information and resources you do have.

Spotlight On: [Fill in the blank] Foods
Gluten

Celiac disease is an autoimmune disorder that leads to damage in the small intestine upon consumption of gluten. It is estimated to affect 1 percent of people worldwide.[15] Even if you don't have celiac disease specifically, many people suffer from non-celiac gluten sensitivity (NCGS). People with NCGS experience symptoms similar to those of celiac disease that resolve when gluten is removed from the diet. However, they do not test positive for celiac disease. Excess inflammation can interfere with your ability to get pregnant, and gluten is a common culprit for causing gut inflammation. Here's what I would say: if you are concerned about your sensitivity to gluten, cut it out of your diet for at least three weeks, and see how you look and feel. If you feel better without it, consider minimizing your intake going forward. If you don't notice any difference, feel free to keep eating it in moderation.

Dairy

There are three main reactions to dairy: dairy allergy (IgE), dairy sensitivity (IgG), and lactose intolerance. In addition to dairy being a top allergen, it has been estimated that ~70 percent of the population has a diminished ability to digest lactose after infancy.[16] Many people are walking around with lactose intolerance (myself included, much to the dismay of my entire Italian family). The best course of action here is to observe your reaction to dairy. Take it out for a while, and see how you feel. If you can tolerate it, great. If not, reevaluate its place in your diet. If you choose to continue having it, choose clean sources (without hormones and antibiotics) and raw sources, if they are available to you locally.

Soy

If you are going to have soy, I would encourage you to choose only fermented soy (such as miso, natto, tamari, and tempeh) and to consume it in small quantities (no more than two to three ounces per day). In large quantities, it can interfere with your hormone levels, particularly estrogen. Soy should be a condiment, not a main staple of your diet.

Coffee

Research on coffee is mixed. This is where you need to tailor your approach. Studies have shown that large amounts of caffeine (five to six cups per day) can increase time to pregnancy and increase miscarriage risk.[17] The impact of less caffeine isn't as clear.

According to GrowBaby Health, women whose daily coffee consumption in pre-pregnancy exceeded four servings, or 400 mg, experienced increased risk of miscarriage compared to women who had no coffee to half a serving of coffee per day. Interestingly, drinking decaffeinated coffee at more than three servings daily was also associated with an increased risk of miscarriage, suggesting a factor at play beyond caffeine levels. Similarly, men whose daily coffee consumption exceeded four servings had increased sperm DNA damage and significantly lower sperm concentration.[18]

Current recommendations from ACOG are to limit caffeine intake to 200 mg daily in preconception and pregnancy to decrease the risk of miscarriage and low birthweight; similar precautions can be taken to improve sperm parameters and decrease sperm oxidative damage in males.[19]

If you have anxiety or high cortisol levels, I would also encourage you to limit coffee consumption. Otherwise, one to two cups per day should be fine, ideally *with food* to minimize the potential negative effects of initiating a cortisol cascade.

Alcohol

Alcohol consumption by either parent during the preconception window can impact the epigenome and increase chronic disease risk.

Studies have shown that alcohol intake during preconception can increase the time to get pregnant as well as increase the risk of miscarriage.[20] In general, it's probably the case that the more alcoholic beverages you consume per week, the longer it is likely to take you to get pregnant. A Harvard Medical School study from 2011 showed that couples undergoing IVF who consumed more than four alcoholic drinks per week each had a 21 percent lower chance of live birth than their peers drinking less than four drinks per week.[21] Some studies have also linked alcohol with ovulatory infertility, but the evidence is not conclusive.[22]

Further, there is evidence that suggests that chronic and/or excessive alcohol intake can negatively impact male reproductive hormones, decreasing testosterone levels and increasing estrogen levels. In males, one study found that sperm concentration, total sperm count, and percentage of spermatozoa with normal morphology were negatively associated with increasing habitual alcohol intake.[23] In other words, the total number of sperm and the proportion of healthy sperm decreased as alcohol intake increased.

Interestingly, in several animal studies, we see that this negative impact is compounded if diabetes is also present. Alcohol consumption in diabetic mice can intensify sperm chromatin/DNA damage, and alcohol further deteriorates sexual dysfunction in diabetic rats.[24] Diabetes + excess alcohol consumption = bad news for sperm.

And it's not just sperm that's affected! High alcohol use in males can impact a baby's life well into the future. According to GrowBaby Health, "Aside from fertility concerns, there is data to suggest that paternal drinking during the preconception period affects behavior, development, and gene expression in the following generations of their offspring."[25]

Your ability to process alcohol is connected to your overall health and lifestyle, as well as your blood sugar management and detox capacity. If you want to be extra conservative, take it out completely. Otherwise, one to two servings of alcohol per week for most females and two to three servings per week for males is probably fine (preferably wine or spirits rather than beer or mixed drinks since the detoxification burden and blood sugar impact is most favorable).

Spotlight On: Blood Sugar Regulation

Blood sugar regulation is a key part of hormonal function. Hormones are all intimately connected and interdependent. Too much sugar leads to too much insulin. Too much insulin leads to too much cortisol and too much testosterone. Too much cortisol depletes estrogen and progesterone. Too much insulin and too much cortisol lead to excess body fat. Excess body fat leads to too much estrogen. And the cycle continues.

Given this cascade, good hormonal balance starts with good blood sugar balance—and good blood sugar balance starts with diet. To encourage optimal blood sugar balance:

- Minimize sugar in all forms.
- Opt for slow carbs (such as whole grains, legumes, and starchy vegetables).
- Pair carbs with protein and fat.
- Eat real food.

I have outlined this in the fertility diet section; however, it bears repeating because it is such a fundamental piece of fertility and is a key part of regulating your menstrual cycle.

If you suspect that you may have blood sugar issues, a continuous glucose monitor may be a helpful tool for monitoring and modifying your food practices to optimize your blood sugar. Please see *9monthsisnotenough.com/bookresources* for additional resources.

Spotlight On: Methylation Support

Methylation is the process by which methyl groups attach to other molecules. Methylation informs many diverse processes in your body: eliminating toxins, including excess estrogen; making neurotransmitters and white blood cells; and generating energy. According to *Younger You* by Dr. Kara Fitzgerald, "Methylation is also required to produce DNA, repair DNA, and—via DNA methylation—control DNA expression."[26] This means that DNA methylation determines which genes get turned on or off and to what extent. We want to support healthy DNA methylation levels because it plays a crucial role in epigenetic expression. Basically, adding a methyl group to a DNA strand (hypermethylation) modulates a gene down, whereas removing methyl groups (hypomethylation) turns a gene on. Dr. Fitzgerald continues, "You want your DNA methylation to be working in such a way that your good genes (those that suppress tumor growth, say) are on and your bad genes (for inflammation, as an example) are generally off." Ultimately, "DNA methylation is the…most impactful of the epigenetic mechanisms and plays a key role in all the major chronic diseases of our time."[27] Of course, as we now know, this can also impact our children's predisposition toward or away from chronic disease.

The punch line is that these methylation processes can be modulated largely by diet and lifestyle. With regard to diet specifically, methyl donors such as folate and vitamin B12 are the nutrients that the body uses to create methyl groups. Methylation adaptogens (e.g., beets, liver, turmeric, rosemary, green tea, cruciferous vegetables), on the other hand, help to ensure that methylation stays appropriately balanced. This is a nuanced topic, so for more juicy details, I suggest Dr. Kara Fitzgerald's groundbreaking book, *Younger You*.

Spotlight On: Popular Diets That Can Interfere with Fertility

Just as we may adopt different fashion styles during different phases of our life, we can also consider adopting different dietary approaches based on our life stage. What's appropriate for one stage of your life may not be appropriate for others, and that is true of many of the popular dietary trends out there when it comes to the pre-pregnancy and pregnancy periods.

Let's look at three diets that may seem healthy but are not the most fertility friendly:

- Low-fat diets
- Vegetarian diets
- Ketogenic diets

Low-Fat Diets Are Linked with Infertility

One groundbreaking study showed that high intake of low-fat dairy foods was associated with infertility. Consumption of lots of low-fat dairy products (e.g., skim milk, o percent fat yogurt) may interfere with regular ovulation, therefore increasing the risk of infertility.[28] This same increased risk of infertility was not seen in study participants who consumed high-fat dairy instead; thus, one can conclude that it was the low-fat component of their diets that contributed to the ovulatory challenges rather than the dairy component of their diets. Further, both animal and human studies have confirmed that low dietary fat intake can interfere with ovulation.[29] Other studies have shown that low-fat diets can lead to reduced estrogen and progesterone levels (this may be helpful for someone trying to avoid breast cancer, as was the case in this study, but less so for someone pursuing fertility).[30] Given this, we may consider that low-fat dairy isn't necessarily the health beacon that it's been hailed to be and could, in fact, be interfering with your efforts to get and stay pregnant.

Vegetarian Diets Are Associated with Lower Overall
Hormone Levels and Increased Menstrual Problems

Females following vegetarian diets have been found to have more menstrual problems, such as irregular periods, heavy periods, and period pain, than their nonvegetarian peers.[31] In small-scale studies, vegetarians were shown to have lower hormone levels than their meat-eating counterparts, and vegetarian diets may induce ovulatory challenges (remember, adequate hormone levels are essential for healthy menstrual cycles).[32] Since the menstrual cycle is the foundation of fertility, menstrual cycle problems are a harbinger of fertility problems down the road.

The reasons for these hormonal discrepancies between vegetarians and nonvegetarians are threefold.

First, as we discussed earlier, you need cholesterol, a form of saturated fat, to make hormones. Granted, plants do contain sterols (the plant equivalent of cholesterol), and your body does make its own cholesterol internally, but your body generally needs more than these two sources to create the optimal level of sex hormones needed for successful reproduction.

Next, certain nutrients are only available or are more bioavailable in animals than they are in plants. For example, despite the many sources of plant protein (such as beans and nuts), animal protein is more easily digested and assimilated than plant protein. Similarly, certain nutrients, such as omega-3 fats and iron, are converted more easily from animal sources than from plant sources. Finally, certain nutrients, such as retinoids (vitamin A), vitamin D, and vitamin B12, only naturally occur in animal foods. All of these nutrients are critical for pre-pregnancy and pregnancy.

Lastly, many vegetarian diets are laden with soy products, which is a phytoestrogen. Phytoestrogens mimic the functions of naturally occurring estrogen in our bodies and can therefore interfere with our natural hormone levels. The last thing we want when trying to get pregnant is to have a large external source of hormones interrupting our own natural supply; that can throw everything out of whack.

The bottom line is that even the most well-intentioned vegan and vegetarian diets are associated with vitamin and mineral deficiencies and therefore can increase the risk of unfavorable fertility and pregnancy outcomes. What might be an acceptable trade-off at other points in your life can become a barrier to success when planning for pregnancy. If you are vegan or vegetarian and are currently having menstrual difficulties, you may want to consider strategically adding some eggs or meat back into your diet. In some cases, it can be really hard to restore a normal menstrual cycle without animal products.

Ketogenic Diets Can Stress Reproductive Function
Too many carbohydrates can contribute to blood sugar and insulin dysregulation issues, which can ultimately interfere with ovulation. On the other hand, too few carbohydrates can signal "scarcity" and "survival" to your body, which then shuttles resources from making your sex hormones to making your stress hormones. When this happens, your body doesn't have adequate sex hormones to menstruate regularly or reproduce. Adequate "slow carbohydrate" intake is necessary to signal to your body that it's safe and stable enough to reproduce.

You did it! You made it through the intricacies of the fertility-friendly diet chapter. Kudos to you.

For some of you, this chapter may have been a refresher on things you already knew or are currently practicing. For others, this may have been completely new content. Wherever your starting point, you're in exactly the right place.

If you're just starting off, you can begin by upgrading your refrigerator and pantry based on the fertility diet guidelines. If you'd like additional tips and resources, you can refer to the resources at *9monthsisnotenough.com/bookresources.*

CHAPTER SUMMARY

- High-quality food is your #1 tool for supporting fertility. The nutritional status of both reproductive partners before conception has profound implications on the long-term health of their children.

- A fertility-friendly diet consists of moderate to high fat intake, moderate complex carbohydrate intake, and moderate protein intake.

- A balanced, whole foods diet is a hormone-friendly diet. Minimize toxins, allergens, and excesses.

- Three popular diets that may seem healthy but are not the most "fertility friendly" are low-fat diets, vegetarian diets, and ketogenic diets.

PRENATAL VITAMINS ARE NECESSARY BUT NOT SUFFICIENT

Start Taking Preconception Supplementation

STATUS CHECK

To get a kick start on understanding what your current nutrition status is, we can look at lab work, including:

- Blood Status (CBC, Ferritin)
- Nutrient Status (Folate, Omega-3/Omega 6 Index, Vitamin B12, Vitamin D)

These tests give us a sense of how you are digesting and assimilating certain key nutrients. If levels are found to be low for any of these nutrients, they are usually easily addressable through dietary changes and/or supplementation.

As we saw in the Introduction, if you've been to your ob-gyn and shared with them that you are planning to get pregnant in the near future, they probably said something to the effect of, "Great! Start taking a prenatal vitamin."

I couldn't agree more that taking a prenatal vitamin is an essential part of pregnancy preparation. That being said, a prenatal vitamin alone is *not enough* for optimal fertility and pregnancy health anymore. In order to set yourself and your future baby up for success, I've developed the optimal preconception formula for supplementation.

Optimal preconception formula for females:

Prenatal + Fish Oil + Egg Health support

Optimal preconception formula for males:

Multivitamin + Fish Oil + Sperm Health support

To come up with these formulas, I leveraged three sources:

1. **Clinical experience**: After working with more clients than I can count in the clinic and running hundreds of lab tests, I was able to pinpoint the nutrients of concern when clients were struggling to get pregnant…and more importantly, I watched

them conceive as we addressed these nutrient deficiencies and imbalances properly.

2. **Clinical studies**: Despite what mainstream media says, there are tons of studies out there that talk about what nutrients can help improve fertility, as indicated by reduced time to pregnancy and improved pregnancy rates.

3. **Fertility clinic protocols**: Many of the best IVF clinics use targeted supplementation in addition to prescription medications for their in vitro fertilization cycles. I pored over their protocols and the success rates with and without these interventions. I chose to focus on those protocols that showed improved success rates without major side effects. Why should only females or males undergoing fertility treatments have access to supplementation that can benefit all individuals trying to conceive?

The bottom line is this: research shows that couples who take fertility-supportive supplements *get pregnant faster and have healthier pregnancies.*

FAQ: BUT WAIT! WHY IS IT NECESSARY TO SUPPLEMENT MY FERTILITY DIET?

Diet is your first line of defense when it comes to supporting fertility. However, even if you have the best diet in the world, you should still consider supplementation as insurance against gaps in the diet, especially during times of increased need such as pregnancy. The act of giving birth alone has been compared to the physical demands of a full marathon, never mind the previous nine months of building and carrying a growing baby.

Even if you have the best intentions, it's hard to eat a balanced diet *all* the time. Even if you succeed most of the time, it's still challenging to get all your nutrient needs met. Dr. Mark Hyman, founder of The UltraWellness Center and best-selling author, sums this up well:

> We evolved eating wild foods that contained dramatically higher levels of all vitamins, minerals, and essential fats. Because of depleted soils, industrial farming, and hybridization techniques, the animals and vegetables we eat have fewer nutrients. Processed factory-made foods have no nutrients. The total burden of environmental toxins, lack of sunlight, and chronic stress leads to higher nutrient needs.
>
> This doesn't even take into account that our own bodies don't always fully digest and assimilate the incredible nutrients we give it due to suboptimal gut function (from incomplete chewing, low stomach acid, stress, etc.). Given this, eating a balanced diet alone isn't enough anymore. We have to do more, and supplementation can really help here, especially during such a critical window as pre-pregnancy and pregnancy.[1]

Furthermore, despite what most magazines will tell you, nutrient needs before and during pregnancy are not just about folate. Folate is critical for pregnant women and women planning to conceive, but the folate discussion crowds out discussion of all of the other nutrients that are essential for a baby's early development.

For example, in babies:

- Low maternal vitamin D status is linked with autism and attention deficit hyperactivity disorder (ADHD).[2]
- Low maternal vitamin B and zinc status have been associated with cleft lip and palate.[3]
- Maternal copper deficiency and zinc deficiency can both lead to intrauterine growth restriction.

And for mom:

- Low maternal status of vitamin D, selenium, zinc, and omega-3s has been associated with postpartum depression.[4]
- Maternal vitamin A deficiency is associated with increased risk of anemia.[5]

All of these micronutrients (vitamins and minerals) are important to ensure the health of your baby and to reinforce your own health. Both a balanced diet *and* targeted supplementation are foundational to make sure that you are getting all these vital nutrients.

The bottom line is that diet is nonnegotiable, but it's not enough. You need targeted, high-quality supplementation as well to adequately support preconception, pregnancy, and postpartum.

THE PRECONCEPTION
SUPPLEMENTATION FORMULA

Here is what I recommend for optimal fertility.

Prenatal Vitamin

A prenatal vitamin is basically a multivitamin with increased focus on certain nutrients, such as folate and iron, that are particularly relevant for the demands of pregnancy.

Why You Need It

The majority of reproductive-age women are micronutrient deficient, meaning they do not have adequate levels of key vitamins and minerals. Nutrient deficiencies can cause problems both getting pregnant and carrying a pregnancy to term, as well as affect your baby's future health trajectory.[6] We always hear about folate in the context of pregnancy, but did you know that adequate folate levels matter for egg development too?

Specifically, when it comes to fertility, prenatal vitamins have been shown to help restore ovulation, boost egg quality, and reduce miscarriage risk. Keep in mind this is what we already know. Preliminary research also suggests that preconception supplementation may reduce the risk of autism and other learning disabilities.[7] I imagine there are many other benefits that we haven't even quantified yet.

Why You Need to Supplement It

A prenatal vitamin is an essential part of pregnancy preparation because in today's society, it's hard to get all the nutrients you need from food alone. Our nutrient needs are higher (given increased stress and toxin loads), and our nutrient sources are lower (given highly processed foods and lower nutrient density of our soil and, therefore, our food). Moreover, pregnancy increases the demand for many nutrients. You need a comprehensive array of micronutrients (vitamins and minerals) to ensure the health of your baby and reinforce your own health. The best way to ensure that is with a high-quality diet *plus* high-quality micronutrient supplementation.

Fish Oil Supplement

Fish oil supplements are concentrated forms of the fatty acid compounds found in certain fish, such as salmon and sardines. Fish oil contains two omega-3 fats called docosahexaenoic acid (DHA) and eicosapentaenoic acid (EPA). Because fish oil is such a critical component of prenatal health, it's being added to many prenatal vitamin formulas.

Why You Need It

Omega-3 fats are essential for both mom and baby. For mom, consumption of cold-water fatty fish and supplementation with fish oil is anti-inflammatory and immunomodulatory. Both inflammation and immune system reactivity can affect a potential pregnancy, so addressing these components is essential for fertility. For baby, omega-3 fats support their brain, eye, and central nervous system development. Because of this, studies have shown that "maternal DHA intake…can enhance visual acuity, hand and eye co-ordination, attention, problem solving and information processing."[8] DHA is also a key component of all cell membranes, which helps to ensure good structural integrity of cells. Studies have found that high maternal intake of fish is associated with a reduction in infant risk for allergic diseases such as eczema and asthma.[9]

Why You Need to Supplement It

Getting adequate levels of EPA and DHA requires special consideration because our body cannot produce either directly. Our intake of EPA and DHA must come from food sources (either directly from fatty fish or converted from foods rich in alpha-linolenic acid or ALA, another omega-3 fat, such as flax or chia seeds) or through supplementation. Most people are not eating fatty fish several times per week, and the conversion from ALA is quite low (less than 15 percent), so supplementation is often necessary to achieve optimal levels, particularly as requirements increase materially during pregnancy.

If you already happen to be eating at least thirty-six ounces of fish per week (e.g. six 6 oz servings), you're getting optimal amounts of EPA and DHA through your diet and likely do not need to take a fish oil supplement. If that is the case, however, I would encourage you to make sure that you are consuming low-mercury fish (e.g., salmon, sardines). See the resources page at *9monthsisnotenough.com/bookresources* for low-mercury fish guides.

If you are vegan or vegetarian, I would still *highly recommend* a fish oil supplement since it is significantly more bioavailable to your body. If you are not comfortable with that, I'd suggest trying an algae-based supplement as an alternative.

Egg Health Supplement

An egg health supplement is predominantly a mitochondrial support supplement. Mitochondria are the energy centers of our cells, and they are particularly relevant for cell division in the early stages of pregnancy.

Why You Need It

Your egg cells are the most mitochondrially dense cells in the entire body, which means they are most susceptible to mitochondrial toxins (e.g., high-sugar diets, unrelenting stress) and most receptive to mitochondrial support (e.g., diverse fruit and vegetable intake, targeted supplementation). Because our current environment is such a drain on egg health and because women are having children later in life, taking an egg health supplement is important to support optimal fertility.

Oxidative stress is involved in the "age-related" decline in fertility. We can blunt the effects of this decline by supporting the production of cellular energy necessary to drive the biological processes involved in egg maturation, providing antioxidant protection to metabolically active eggs and potentially supporting the hormonal environment of the ovaries.

SpectraCell, a nutrient testing company, found that "overwhelming evidence suggests that infertility issues stem from low antioxidant status. Deficiencies in vitamins C and E, zinc, copper, magnesium, folate as well as the powerful antioxidant cysteine have been linked to infertility. In many cases, targeted repletion is very beneficial with fertility and related issues like polycystic ovary syndrome, which are also strongly linked to oxidative stress."[10] Because of this, antioxidants are powerful nutrients to support mitochondria and, in turn, egg health.

Why You Need to Supplement It

Many antioxidants can be produced by the body. However, the rigors of daily living cause oxidative stress and often use up much of our antioxidant stores. Because the antioxidant levels we need for optimal fertility are high and because our antioxidant stores tend to be depleted, supplementation is the best way to ensure that you have adequate levels for fertility.

Supplementation for Males

This may come as no surprise, but much of the same logic applies to supplementation for males. As we've discussed in previous chapters, both sperm quantity and sperm quality are important for conception. The more sperm you have, the better the chances that one of them will be vital enough to fertilize the egg, and sperm need to be in tip-top shape (able to swim fast and be the right shape) to reach and penetrate the egg.

Much like egg cells, sperm cells are uniquely sensitive to free radical damage. The cell membrane of sperm contains high amounts of fats that are easily damaged by free radicals. Unfortunately, sperm do not have the antioxidant mechanisms to combat the overwhelming number of free radicals they are exposed to on a daily basis. As a result, it is important to support sperm health with omega-3 fats to fortify their cellular structure and antioxidants to combat the oxidative damage from free radicals.

Certain antioxidants (e.g., Vitamins C and E, CoQ10), amino acids (e.g., L-Carnitine, L-Arginine), and vitamins and minerals (e.g., zinc, selenium, Vitamin B12), have all been shown to improve sperm parameters. Studies have shown a statistically significant improvement in sperm count, progressive motility, and normal morphology after three months of sperm health supplements, in addition to significant improvements in DNA fragmentation.

Often, a traditional multivitamin does not contain the targeted nutrients necessary to optimize sperm health, which is why an additional sperm health supplement is recommended. In addition, fish oil supplements with EPA and DHA have been shown to help maintain the integrity of sperm cell membranes and sperm motility.

The bottom line is that men need preconception supplementation too. Don't make your reproductive partner do all of the work. It's important that you are doing your part to reach your fertility and family goals.

There you have it—the ultimate preconception formula for supplementation!

Spotlight On: Gut Support

A conversation about supplementation would not be complete without discussing gut function.

Probiotics have become so popular in the past few years because most of us have significantly impaired digestive function from limited microbial amounts and diversity. This is because of the rampant use of antibiotics, high levels of stress, highly processed foods, and so forth. Because of this, our bodies are not getting the materials they need (namely, lots of different sources of fiber) to generate bacterial balance and diversity. This often results in impaired gut function and, therefore, a lower-functioning immune system.

However, gut support involves more than popping a probiotic. The foundation of gut health involves fortifying your entire gut barrier. According to Dr. Sarah Rahal, founder of ARMRA, "A healthy mucosal barrier is one that is in balance—allowing the body to absorb essential nutrients while also keeping out harmful substances from everything we breathe, eat, and drink."[11]

Much of the gut health conversation over the past several years has focused on the microbiome. However, the gut mucosal barrier has four different layers (Gut Cell Barrier, Mucous Layer, Microbiome, and Immune Cells and Antibodies), and the microbiome is only one of them.

Comprehensive gut support can include things that improve the microbial balance in your gut (e.g., prebiotics, probiotics), things that restore your gut lining (e.g., certain growth factors or nutrients), and things that improve the function of your digestion or assimilation (e.g., enzymes).

Why You Need It

Digestive health is the foundation of overall health and, in particular, immune health. Unfortunately, as we've discussed many times, our modern environment erodes our gut function. Dr. Rahal explains:

Each day, our bodies are bombarded by a host of disruptive things that weaken this line of defense. Air pollutants, pesticides in the food and water supply, medications, stress hormones, refined carbohydrates, processed food, and micronutrient deficiencies, among other factors, disrupt the architecture and make the barrier more penetrable. This makes it easier for harmful particles to get inside, including viruses, bacteria, molds, allergens, and environmental toxins...not only can these exposures make us ill, they can also activate the immune system inappropriately and trigger inflammation. This leads to a host of modern health issues such as: autoimmune conditions, allergies, weight gain, bloating, digestive issues, mental fog, sleep disturbances, depression and anxiety...without healthy immune barriers, we are more vulnerable to threats that negatively impact our health and performance.[12]

A balanced gut, on the other hand, is the foundation of vibrant health. It helps with nutrient digestion and absorption, toxin elimination, and pathogen defense, among many other things. Another thing to keep in mind is that your baby inherits your microbiome, so the more you nourish your microbiome before and during pregnancy, the more robust your child's microbiome will be.

Why You May Need to Supplement It

The ideal way to nourish your gut is through food—with fiber, probiotic-rich foods (foods that contain live bacteria or active cultures like kefir, kimchi, sauerkraut, and kombucha), prebiotic foods (foods that feed bacteria such as asparagus, onion, garlic, and leeks), and nutrient-dense foods that repair your gut lining.

If you are going to use probiotics, it is recommended to cycle them—take a probiotic supplement (with live bacteria), and then eat prebiotic foods to feed the growth of the bacteria that you just implanted in your digestive tract. Rinse, repeat. Probiotic supplements can be a great way to infuse a large amount of beneficial bacteria into your system quickly (a recolonization of bacteria in your gut). However, if you take probiotics alone without upgrading your diet, particularly with prebiotic foods, you aren't taking full advantage of the probiotic supplement. Probiotics and prebiotics work together for a happy gut.

In addition, it is important to reconstitute the lining of your gut since it is being broken down by so many things on a daily basis. Certain essential nutrients such as zinc and vitamins A, C, D, and E are all helpful, as are amino acids. Boosters like colostrum, collagen, aloe vera, and glutamine can also be very effective to amplify results.

Supplementation prior to pregnancy makes it easier to get pregnant, increases the likelihood of a healthy pregnancy, and sets the stage for a healthier baby. Unfortunately, not all supplements are created equal, so make sure you choose quality providers. See *9monthsisnotenough.com/ bookresources* for some of my favorite brands. This will ensure that you are getting the right form of the vitamin at the right dosage with minimal additives and fillers.

In addition to the supplements listed above, which are recommended for all individuals planning to conceive, there may be additional supplementation relevant to your personal situation. For example:

- Myo-inositol has some good evidence to support its use in females with PCOS.[13]
- If you are over the age of thirty-five, both DHEA and progesterone can be considered.
- If you are vegan or vegetarian, you may need more of certain nutrients (e.g., vitamin B12, iron).
- If you travel a lot or really want to eat more greens but just don't manage to, a high-quality greens powder might be a good option to consider.
- For individuals with low vitamin D, an incremental vitamin D supplement beyond what is in your prenatal or multivitamin may be prudent (I align with the functional ranges of ~50–75 ng/mL vitamin D, as the traditional reference ranges seem to be too low for optimal health and fertility).
- For females with anemia, supplemental iron may also be necessary.
- If you are dealing with a chronic disease or have recently undergone surgery, you may need additional protein.

Supplementation can be the Wild West, with so many options to choose from and such a wide variety of quality; however, targeted supplementation can be incredibly effective to amplify your health goals when used in the right dose at the right time.

CHAPTER SUMMARY

- Diet is non-negotiable, but it's not enough. You need targeted, high-quality supplementation as well to adequately support preconception, pregnancy, and postpartum.

- Men need preconception supplementation too.

- The optimal preconception formula = Prenatal Multivitamin + Fish Oil + Egg/Sperm Health support

- Additional supplementation may be warranted based on your pre-pregnancy wellness baseline.

MOVE IT TO GROOVE IT

Adopt a Fertility-Friendly Movement Plan

- Metabolic Status
  - Blood Sugar Management (Glucose, Hemoglobin A1C, Insulin)
  - Cholesterol Metabolism (Lipid Panel)

Study after study has shown that exercise is a positive contributor to overall health. Every magazine headline reinforces this message, as do healthcare professionals and the entire fitness industry. At this point, I think most of us would acknowledge that exercise is good for us.

However, when I was working as a personal trainer, I found that whether my clients exercised consistently or not was predicated on two things:

1. The why: What inspired them to work out?
2. The how: Was it feasible and, for the most part, enjoyable?

Those two topics are exactly what we are going to cover in this chapter.

Rather than spending time telling you that exercise is good for you, I want to spend time talking about how exercise impacts fertility, as well as differentiating between how much and what type of exercise is ideal to support fertility. Hopefully, this influences both the reasons behind your motivation to exercise (the why) and your ability to find things that work for you (the how).

Please note: In most cases throughout this chapter, I will use the word movement instead of exercise. I've worked with hundreds of women, and I find that the term exercise can have a negative connotation. Exercise can be seen as punishing and foreboding for many people, and that's not the association I am espousing here. Movement is a more all-encompassing term. Movement can be gentle, or it can be more active, depending on your desire and ability. It can also include daily movement practices (e.g., walking) as well as intentional exercise practices (e.g., interval training, weight training). If you already have a great relationship with exercise, then kudos to you! Rock on. If not, I hope to provide a more inspiring approach to help you get started.

HOW MOVEMENT IMPACTS FERTILITY

I'll start with the key takeaway: regular movement practices can support ovulation, egg quality, and a healthy uterine environment, all of which improve your chances of a healthy conception. Movement has been shown to have the same positive effects on sperm quality.[1] Here's how:

- **Movement supports detoxification.** As we discussed in Chapter 9, regular movement practices support detoxification primarily through two of the major detox organs: skin (sweating) and lungs (breathing). Sweating helps to eliminate toxins from the body through your largest detox organ, your skin. Deep breathing helps dispel stale air from the lungs and replaces it with fresh oxygen to support detoxification processes. Certain exercises, like jumping rope, can also stimulate your lymphatic system, which supports the expulsion of waste products from your body.

- **Movement improves circulation.** It increases blood flow, which brings oxygen and nutrients to your organs, including your reproductive organs. It helps to get rid of any stagnation such as blood clots. This may also help to clear any adhesions and blockages in the reproductive area.

- **Movement helps improve insulin sensitivity.** As we saw in Chapter 12, blood sugar management is a key factor in fertility. When blood sugar is not balanced, it can cause a negative hormonal cascade that ultimately interferes with ovulation. Remember, ovulating regularly is a foundational step to getting pregnant. Studies have shown that exercise has both long-term and short-term effects on insulin sensitivity.[2] Single exercise sessions produce immediate effects, lasting up to seventy-two hours post-exercise, while regular exercise sessions have been shown to produce long-term, chronic improvement in insulin sensitivity. This may be one of the reasons studies have shown that exercise is associated with a reduced risk of ovulatory infertility (i.e., infertility due to irregular or absent ovulation).

- **Movement has been shown to have great psychological benefits**. It helps manage stress levels and regulate mood. It also modulates cortisol levels. Unchecked cortisol levels can interfere with our sex hormones and our fertility.

- **Movement helps reduce inflammation.** Ongoing inflammation (e.g., from high sugar, processed foods, stress, sleep deprivation) can interfere with your ability to get pregnant, so it's important to keep inflammation in check.

- **Movement supports a healthy immune system.** An underactive immune system can make you susceptible to a variety of pathogens (e.g., bacteria, viruses). An overactive immune system (as in autoimmune disease) can interfere with your ability to maintain a pregnancy. You want your immune system to be vigilant but discerning.

All of these factors contribute to increased circulation and nutrient flow to your ovaries (and eggs) and uterus in females and testes (and sperm) in males. Well-functioning circulation brings in the good stuff (e.g., nutrients) and takes away the bad stuff (e.g., toxins). This, in turn, can improve your egg health and uterine environment.

The same logic applies for males. Research indicates that moderate exercise increases sperm production.[3] In addition, regular exercise has also been shown to improve sperm motility (apparently, the more your body moves and grooves, the more your sperm do too!).[4]

HOW MOVEMENT AFFECTS PREGNANCY, POSTPARTUM, AND BEYOND

Now that you know how movement affects fertility, it's also important to discuss how starting a movement practice now sets you up well for pregnancy, postpartum, and beyond. You are about to embark on quite a physically demanding period of your life. Rather than merely surviving it, I want to set you up to thrive.

Most people intuitively recognize that pregnancy is highly physically demanding, but not many people talk about the real implications of these demands. In fact, for many people, pregnancy, childbirth, and early motherhood is the most physically demanding period of their lives.

During pregnancy, there are significant physiological stresses put on the body. Your hormones shift. Your cardio-respiratory system function expands. Your musculoskeletal system changes to accommodate your growing baby. The average pregnant woman gains between twenty-five and thirty-five pounds in the span of four to six months.

Then, after the rigorous demands of carrying a pregnancy for nine months, the birth itself is physically demanding. Then, being a new mom is physically demanding (e.g., nonstop physical demands including breastfeeding, lifting and carrying a baby, chasing around after a growing baby, and minimal sleep).

Pronatal Fitness, one of the leaders in prenatal and postnatal fitness, sums it up well:

The motherhood journey places a tremendous amount of stress on the body—from the physical changes of pregnancy, to the marathon of childbirth, followed by the non-stop physical 24/7 demands of infant care. It is truly one of life's greatest athletic events, and we believe in training for it as such.[5]

I love this approach—thinking of pregnancy as an "athletic event" is an amazing reframe. Rather than being overwhelmed by what's to come, it also means that we can treat pregnancy and birth as an athletic event that you can prepare for, much like you would prepare for a 5K race or a triathlon.

The status quo for many females (who often haven't ever been told there's another option) is to really struggle with their bodies during and post-pregnancy. Nearly 50 percent of women gain more than the recommended amount of weight during pregnancy. They constantly feel tired and lethargic. They don't feel very strong or fit. Then, they struggle with their post-baby body.

My message to you is this: it doesn't have to be this way.

Yes, there are some inevitabilities—you will gain weight to accommodate a growing baby. You will undergo hormonal shifts. You will have to modify your previous activities to account for your new body and its needs. *However, the stronger and fitter you are, the better you will be at mitigating the effects of the weight gain and all the other physical changes.* Ideally, the goal is to enjoy pregnancy, not merely to endure it.

Doing that takes preparation! Do you sense a theme going on here?

When you prepare in advance, pregnancy is easier. Birth is easier. Postpartum is easier. Notice I didn't say *easy?*

Being a mom will be a lot easier (and more fun) when you are healthy and fit. Moreover, children born to healthier moms are more likely to be healthy themselves. Children born to fitter moms have also been shown to score higher on intelligence and language tests in adolescence. Beyond physical benefits, fitness confers cognitive benefits for your children as well.

Here's the evidence, according to GrowBaby Health:

- Move for your health: Moderate physical exercise during pregnancy has been shown to reduce the incidence and magnitude of depression, reduce the frequency of gestational diabetes in overweight or obese women, and minimize the risk of hypertension and excessive weight gain in pregnancy. Furthermore, exercise has been shown to reduce delivery and neonatal complications.

- Move for your baby's health: "Children of mothers who exercised in pregnancy...are born with more mature brains, even showing [improved cognitive] performance in the children of women who exercised regularly throughout pregnancy. There is also an association between mothers who exercise during pregnancy and lowered risk of low birth weight."[6]

The optimal time to improve maternal fitness is *before* pregnancy. Preconception training pays off with a better and smoother journey through pregnancy, postpartum, and beyond. And it has clear and compelling benefits for your future baby!

Now that you know *why* movement is important for fertility, pregnancy, and postpartum, it's time to talk about *how* to exercise for fertility.

EXERCISE QUANTITY: THE DOSE MAKES THE POISON

You're probably tired of hearing me talk about the Goldilocks principle (not too little, not too much, right in the middle) by now, but it strikes again with regard to exercise!

Not Too Little

You may have heard the comment that "sitting is the new smoking." Maybe that's a bit dramatic, but it's not something to be overlooked. According to the Mayo Clinic:

Research has linked sitting for long periods of time with a number of health concerns. They include obesity and a cluster of conditions—increased blood pressure, high blood sugar, excess body fat around the waist and unhealthy cholesterol levels—that make up metabolic syndrome.[7]

These increased risks are *independent of other cardiac risk factors* like smoking and high blood pressure.

Remember, anything that affects your overall health is also likely to affect your fertility. More importantly, "spending a few hours a week at the gym or otherwise engaged in moderate or vigorous activity doesn't seem to significantly offset the risk." In other words, working out a few times a week (even at a high intensity) cannot offset sitting all day long.

In males, sitting for long periods of time may be associated with an increased risk for varicoceles (enlarged veins in the scrotum). Varicoceles can decrease testosterone production in the testes and, in some cases, cause azoospermia, or the complete absence of sperm in the ejaculate. For these reasons, varicoceles can profoundly impact male fertility.

Because of this, it's not just about adding exercise into your daily routine. It's about sitting less *and* moving more overall.

PRECONCEPTION TIP

Hack your environment to encourage more movement. A few simple suggestions are standing desks, balance balls, and rebounders (indoor trampolines). Fun fact: you burn 30 percent more calories when you're standing than when you're sitting.

Not Too Much

Exercise is a stressor. While some stressors are good for us and can force us to adapt and get stronger, excessive intense exercise can exacerbate stress to levels that are incompatible with optimal fertility.

Certain types of exercise, in particular, are known to increase cortisol levels. Short-term, increased cortisol isn't necessarily a bad thing, but if you already have an issue with elevated cortisol or if you are choosing sports that chronically elevate your cortisol levels, you may want to reconsider. For example, HIIT raises cortisol levels in the short term, while distance running can raise cortisol levels long term.[8] Because of this, studies have shown that ongoing, vigorous exercise (e.g., running, cycling) has been associated with infertility.[9]

The key with exercise is to not overdo it because excessive exercise can make it tougher to get pregnant. Everyone is different, so let your body be the guide as to what is "too much" for you. If you consistently feel drained after exercising, you're probably doing too much. If you're sore for days after a workout, you probably pushed too hard. For females, if you are missing periods, that may be a sign to pare things back on the exercise front.

Right in the Middle

Aim for the "sweet spot" where exercise is challenging but invigorating.

What's the sweet spot? It's a bit different for everyone, depending on your current starting point and previous athletic experience, but here are the guidelines we have to work with:

- A landmark study showed that *thirty minutes of physical activity per day* was associated with decreased risk of ovulatory infertility.[10]

- The American College of Obstetricians and Gynecologists recommends aerobic and strength training *before, during, and after* pregnancy. They suggest twenty to thirty minutes per day of moderate-intensity exercise on most days of the week.[11]

- A study in *Obstetrics and Gynecology* found that women who exercised thirty minutes or more daily had a reduced risk of infertility due to ovulation disorders.[12]

In summary, I think we can safely say that around thirty minutes of physical activity most days of the week can help support your fertility goals.

Now that we know how to think about movement, let's talk about what types of exercise to consider.

EXERCISE TYPE: MIX AND MATCH

I'd put exercise into three main categories: cardiovascular, strength, and mobility. Of course, there is overlap between these three areas, but we can talk about them in these broad buckets.

Cardiovascular exercise includes activities like running, spinning, swimming, high-intensity interval training (HIIT), long-distance race training, sports, and dance.

Quite simply, better cardiovascular health = better metabolic health.

Cardiovascular exercise helps manage insulin levels better, improve blood pressure, and improve lung function, all of which are beneficial when trying to get pregnant. Better cardiovascular function also translates into an easier pregnancy and delivery—you have better endurance/stamina, don't tire as easily, and recover more quickly. Doesn't that sound nice?

Strength training includes activities like weight lifting, resistance training (e.g., resistance bands, TRX), and weight-bearing exercises (e.g., walking). Having good muscle development, including a high strength-to-weight ratio, is particularly helpful during pregnancy.

Mobility practices include activities like yoga and Pilates. Some experts believe that certain yoga poses can increase blood flow to your pelvis, support detoxification, and release muscle tension, all of which can enhance baby-making ability. Pilates is great for developing core and back strength, both of which are beneficial for pregnancy.

Ideally, you want to mix and match between the three categories of exercise to get the most diverse benefits. If you already have a strong cardio practice, maybe sprinkle in some strength training once or twice per week. If you over-index on strength training, maybe incorporate some mobility work. If you are squarely focused on mobility, maybe upgrade the intensity a bit with cardio or strength bursts. That being said, I like to operate in the real world, not in the ideal world. For this reason, I would suggest choosing the activities you enjoy doing the most (even if that isn't perfectly balanced across all three categories).

The key here is to explore enough different modalities that you can find something that lights you up. Exercise should be challenging, but invigorating. If something doesn't feel good in your body, then don't do it! Keep searching until you find something that you look forward to doing. If you do what feels good to you, you are more likely to stick with it. For the most part, consistency/frequency of movement is more important than intensity of movement.

Please note: If you have high cortisol levels or adrenal fatigue, you will want to minimize intense cardio sessions since this only exacerbates that condition. I've seen many women in my clinic who are doing several spinning classes a week or long-distance running sessions, and they completely lose their menstrual cycle as a result. I hate to be the bearer of bad news, but you may need to lay off the intense cardio sessions for a bit to signal to your body that you're not running from a lion. You don't need to eliminate exercise, of course, but you may need to shift the types and quantity of exercise that you do for a bit.

CHAPTER SUMMARY

- The benefits of movement are multifactorial. It supports detoxification, circulation, insulin regulation, mindset, inflammation levels, and immunity.

- You can treat pregnancy as an athletic event that you can prepare for.

- Exercise is good for fertility, pregnancy, and your future baby.

- Spending less time sitting overall is a great starting point.

- With exercise, the dose makes the poison. Too little or too much exercise can interfere with fertility.

GET YOUR MENTAL GAME IN ORDER

Optimize Sleep and Stress

Cortisol gives us a peek into how your body is adapting to stressors in your life. We also want to look at inflammatory markers, since inflammation has been associated with mood disorders. When we are stressed, our nutrient needs increase, and we don't digest and assimilate nutrients as well, so checking nutrient status can be helpful. Stress can also affect blood sugar regulation. In addition, stress can impact immunity, and issues with immunity can increase stress. The effects of stress are far-reaching and can cascade through every one of our bodily systems.

ave you ever heard of a couple who's been trying to get pregnant for years, and then they initiate an adoption process and miraculously get pregnant? Or a couple who struggled to conceive their first child and eventually got pregnant through IVF only to conceive naturally—with twins—the second time around? The stress response could be one of the reasons. So that really unhelpful advice to "just relax" when it comes to trying to conceive—well, as patronizing as it may be, there is some wisdom to it. It's actually grounded in science.

Your sex hormones and your stress hormones are in the same biochemical pathway. As a reminder, your body will always prioritize survival over procreation.

Practically speaking, this means that when we are constantly stressed (whether from a long commute, regimented marathon training, or significant financial obligations), our bodies divert the raw materials needed to make our sex hormones to make our stress hormones instead. Over time, that means that we don't have the necessary sex hormones to get pregnant or sustain a pregnancy.

In females, estrogen and progesterone are the hormones needed for the egg to mature and ovulate, as well as to prepare the uterus for implantation of the fertilized egg. A shortage of progesterone can cause a hormonal imbalance, leading to irregular menstrual cycles and impacting an egg's ability to mature and a fertilized egg's ability to thrive. It can even result in amenorrhea (missed periods altogether).

Further, stress in early pregnancy has been found to result in localized inflammation in the uterus, reduced production of progesterone (which is essential to maintaining early pregnancy), and increased production of adrenaline (which can directly interfere with development of the embryo). In addition, research is now showing that high amounts of stress experienced by the mother during gestation may have adverse outcomes for both the mom and baby and may have lasting consequences that span generations. These implications include higher rates of obesity, diabetes, and cardiovascular disease; increased risk of infertility; and higher rates of mood disorders.[1]

Similarly, in males, stress has been shown to impact sperm health. Elevated, chronic stress levels impact semen volume and semen quality.[2]

This is all to say that high levels of chronic stress can impact your ability to get pregnant, stay pregnant, and have a healthy pregnancy. Similar to how we approach detoxification, we want to minimize as many unnecessary stressors as possible. For those that we can't eliminate, we want to enhance our ability to manage them.

Okay, let's take a step back for a second and demystify the "big bad wolf" commonly known as stress.

WHAT IS STRESS?

Stress is a psychological or physiological response to something perceived as threatening.

A stressor is something that triggers a stress response. There are several types of stressors. When we think of stress, we usually think of *psychological stressors* (e.g., a disagreement with a partner, an overbearing parent, work deadlines). Those can absolutely contribute to our stress load. In addition, there are also *physiological stressors*, such as underlying infections (e.g., STIs, Lyme disease, gum disease), food sensitivities, or overtraining. These are more insidious but can increase stress on the body no less. We tend to over-focus on the psychological stressors and under-focus on the physiological stressors. That's why the advice to "just relax" is insufficient. It's also important to understand that your body can be experiencing stress without you "feeling stressed" per se.

PUBLIC SERVICE ANNOUNCEMENT

In this chapter, we discuss the epidemic of stress that is affecting millions of people. I would be remiss not to mention the epidemic of mental health disorders that are also on the rise. Depression and anxiety are at all-time highs. I am not a mental health expert, so I will keep my comments here short. Two of the best resources that I've found on the topic of mental health are Dr. Kelly Brogan's book, *A Mind of Your Own*, and Johann Hari's book, *Lost Connections*. They are fairly countercultural to the traditional narrative around the source of and remedy for mental health. They are also much more holistic in approach, which is why I find them refreshing. Feel free to check them out if that resonates with you too.

WHAT HAPPENS WHEN WE GET STRESSED?

Any acute or chronic stressor is perceived as a threat to our survival, and our body responds accordingly. When you are stressed, the following cascade of events happens in your body:

- Adrenaline and cortisol increase.
- Blood thickens and coagulates.
- Bladder and bowels evacuate.
- Vision narrows.
- Digestion shuts down.
- Immune system function downregulates.

All nonessential functions (e.g., digestion, immunity) are shut down in order to focus resources on your ability to survive (e.g., heightened senses, ability to run faster/climb higher). Your body is trying to protect you. When our main stressor was running from a lion, this was a finely tuned response. We needed all hands on deck to handle a predator, preparing to either fight or flee. In either case, the situation would be over in a matter of minutes. The cocktail of hormones secreted in this scenario were meant to mobilize quickly and then dissipate quickly.

Now, stress means running from your unrelenting boss's demands or your family's unrealistic expectations. Though your boss and your family aren't truly threatening your survival, your primal brain doesn't know that and responds as if they were. This response would be fine if it only lasted a few minutes, as did an encounter with a lion. However, given today's stressors, this cascade of events stays turned on for far longer than it was originally intended to and has become maladaptive for today's "threats." It's an outdated reaction to modern demands. As a result, it can cause a host of health problems, including poor digestion and assimilation of nutrients, elevated blood sugar, and premature aging.

Your body was designed to handle short bursts of intense stress. But when that level of stress becomes your default mode, it can have broader health consequences, including impacting fertility. This chronic stress, or stress that interferes with your ability to function normally over an extended period of time, is becoming a public health crisis. Stress levels are at an all-time high. We are bombarded with a litany of demands on a daily basis—balancing obligations from our family and our career; navigating relationships with our partner, parents, friends, and coworkers; commuting to work; eating on the run; and struggling to get in an extra hour of sleep. We are more stressed and stretched than ever before in human history. Furthermore, as we discussed in Chapter 1, reproductive anxiety is on the rise, and just thinking about getting pregnant has become stressful for many couples. There are so many messages out there that make couples question their ability to get pregnant and to have a healthy baby. This adds stress to an already stressful situation.

The important takeaway is that chronic stress is on the rise and is more problematic for our health than acute stress.

A SLEEP EPIDEMIC

We are also experiencing a sleep epidemic. According to the CDC, 35 percent of Americans are getting less than the recommended seven hours of sleep each night, and according to the National Sleep Foundation, about 35 percent of adults experience difficulty falling asleep or staying asleep.[3] Sleep and stress are intimately connected: lack of sleep increases stress, and stress makes it harder to sleep. Also, circadian rhythms and melatonin levels influence ovulation, which is why your cycles may be irregular while traveling and why females who work the night shift can experience increased fertility challenges. Getting adequate sleep is essential for health and fertility.

I recognize that this is a luxury and certainly hasn't always been the case, but I currently try not to use an alarm clock to wake up most days to ensure that my body gets the rest it needs. I would encourage you to do whatever it takes to optimize your sleep environment to get the rest that your body requires—eye shades, white-noise machines, acupressure mats, weighted blankets, cooling mats, aromatherapy. I've experimented with them all. Sleep hygiene is individual, so find what works best for you. I used to think that good food was my foundational habit, the core habit upon which everything else is built (I am a nutritionist, after all!), but over the years, I have found that good sleep is. It is the domino habit that affects everything else downstream. If I don't sleep well, I am prone to move less, eat less healthily, think less clearly, and be less social. That is not how I want to show up every day, so I am meticulous about my sleep. I would encourage you to try it for a few weeks and see how you feel. Sleep really is the gift that keeps on giving.

HOW TO BE BETTER AT STRESS

Now that we've covered how detrimental chronic stress can be, let's talk about what we can do about it.

Reframe How You Think about Stress

Many people think that they would be happier if there was less stress in their lives. However, research suggests the contrary. People are generally happier when they are busy and engaged with life, even if that means having more responsibility than they would otherwise choose. Kelly McGonigal, author of *The Upside of Stress*, explains, "Rather than being a sign that something is wrong with your life, feeling stressed can be a barometer for how engaged you are in activities and relationships that are personally meaningful."

McGonigal goes on to say that your stress mindset "shapes everything from the emotions you feel during a stressful situation to the way you cope with stressful events. That, in turn, can determine whether you thrive under stress or end up burned out and depressed."[4]

It's not about avoiding stress; it's about managing your perceptions of and reactions to it. If there are certain things that you can't change about your life, reframe them or upgrade them. For example, if you are stressed about a big project at work, focus on how much of a badass you are for being given this opportunity and how appreciative you are. If you are stressed about your morning commute but can't eliminate it right now, upgrade it with an amazing playlist, an uplifting podcast, or a phone call to a friend.

One of the most powerful reframes of stress I've ever heard comes from Emily Fletcher, founder of Ziva Meditation: "Adaptation energy: Your ability to handle a demand or a change of expectation."[5] The goal of meditation or any "stress management" practice is to increase your adaptation energy—your ability to adapt to whatever comes your way. We all juggle many demands on our time, energy, and attention; stress is the negative impact that we allow those demands to have. It is not the demand itself—it is our reaction to it. Even reframing the word "stressor" to "demand" made things lighter for me.

The bottom line is that shifting your mindset from one that avoids anxiety at all costs to a belief that embraces stress as a normal part of life helps you respond to it in more effective ways. Embracing stress can have a positive impact on our mental and physical health if we approach it with the appropriate mindset. And for goodness' sake, don't stress about feeling stressed. Stress is natural and normal... and, at the risk of repeating myself again, unavoidable. It's okay to be stressed; just don't make it your default mode all day, every day.

Identify Sources of "Demand" in Your Life

Think broadly. Here is a starter list to get the juices flowing:

- Finances (e.g., taxes, unpaid bills, unplanned expenses)
- Work (e.g., high-pressure work environment, deadlines, restrictive rules)
- Relationships (e.g., conflict with others, loneliness, not spending enough time with important people in your life)
- Health (e.g., illness, injury, low energy)
- Life events (e.g., promotion, moving, marriage, divorce)
- Lifestyle (e.g., not enough sleep, too much caffeine/ alcohol, poor diet)
- Physical environment (e.g., bright lights, noise, excessive heat or cold, weather, traffic)

Eliminate Any Unnecessary Demands That You Can

Prioritize what really matters to you and let go of worrying about everything else. *The Life-Changing Magic of Not Giving a F*ck* by Sarah Knight is a great thought starter on this topic. Over time, anything that depletes your energy more than it elevates your energy should be eliminated. This may include your commute to work, an underlying infection, an exercise routine you hate, or even a draining relationship.

Manage What You Can't Eliminate

In addition to baseline health practices (like eating a balanced diet, regular exercise/movement, and getting high-quality sleep), mindfulness practices have also been shown to be beneficial for stress reduction—and, in turn, fertility health. A mindfulness practice can reduce the stress you currently experience through your thoughts and feelings, as well as allow you to become better equipped to handle whatever upcoming stress you may face.

Let's look at an analogy for how to think about stress management. In your bank account, there is a monetary reserve. Some weeks, you add to it (savings). Other weeks, you deduct from it (spending). In order to keep a positive balance, you have to do more saving than spending; otherwise, you will deplete your bank account to zero (or even negative). The same is true of your stress account. Some weeks, you add to it (relaxing and rejuvenating). Other weeks, you deduct from it (stressing and complaining). In order to keep a positive balance, you have to do more relaxing and rejuvenating than stressing and complaining. It's all about keeping a positive balance.

Sometimes, identifying ways to contextualize and manage physical or psychological stress can benefit from the help of a skilled practitioner, such as a coach, therapist, acupuncturist, hypnotherapist, or massage therapist. However, there are also many techniques that are essentially free and can be done in the comfort of your own home. These include:

Meditation

There are many different forms of meditation—Transcendental, mindfulness, loving kindness, mantra, guided, and the list goes on. The two that I practice regularly myself are Ziva Meditation by Emily Fletcher and guided meditations by Dr. Joe Dispenza.

Meditation has many recorded benefits, including improved focus and memory, increased optimism, decreased stress and anxiety, improved immune function, reduced blood pressure, more restful sleep, increased energy, and so much more.

One of the biggest benefits of meditation for fertility is that it helps reduce cortisol levels (and we know the havoc that unchecked cortisol can wreak from our mini science class above). High cortisol lowers our sex hormones, so reducing cortisol can help normalize sex hormone levels as a necessary precursor to getting pregnant.

Tapping/EFT (Emotional Freedom Technique)

EFT utilizes the meridian system, which has been used in acupuncture for thousands of years. Instead of needles, you use your fingers to tap on specific points on the face and upper body that mirror some of the acupuncture points. While tapping, you focus on whatever is bothering you and verbally process your feelings about an issue.

For example, you will start by saying, "Even though (I have this fear of x, I have this guilt about y, I'm anxious about z, etc.), I completely love and accept myself." Tapping helps you to release the tension associated with the issue at hand, process the issue in your mind and body, and reduce stress.

It sounds a bit woo-woo for sure, but it is remarkably effective for reducing cortisol levels. According to *The Tapping Solution*, one study showed an average of a 24 percent reduction in cortisol after a one-hour EFT session compared to a much smaller reduction from one hour of talk therapy.[6] That's pretty powerful stuff! If nothing else, it's worth trying.

Gratitude

A regular gratitude practice has been shown to:

- **Improve physical health.** Grateful people report fewer physical ailments, better sleeping habits, and higher vitality than other people.[7] Moreover, grateful people are also more likely to take care of their health.

- **Improve psychological health.** Gratitude increases happiness and reduces depression. It has also been shown to improve people's ability to overcome trauma.

- **Improve prosocial behaviors.** Gratitude increases empathy and reduces social comparisons. Rather than becoming resentful toward people who have better perceived circumstances, grateful people are able to appreciate other people's accomplishments.

It seems incredibly simple, but sometimes the most basic practices win out. What we appreciate appreciates.

Journaling

Journaling can help you process some of the feelings that may come up around your fertility journey, some of which may even be uncovered through the other modalities discussed here. A regular journaling practice can be helpful for you to process thoughts you feel like you can't share with others or even to uncover thoughts you weren't even consciously aware of.

There are lots of different types of journaling. You can get a guided journal with built-in questions or prompts for you to respond to, or you can read a passage in a book and then write about what comes up for you. You can do something called "morning pages" (which *The Artist's Way* describes as three pages of longhand, stream-of-consciousness writing done first thing in the morning).

Take your pick, and write away. No one will see it unless you want them to.

Breathwork

Breathing is something that we do automatically, but deliberate breath practices can be one of the most accessible and powerful practices to adopt for stress management, with benefits for mental, physical, and emotional levels. When you engage in breathwork, you have the ability to shift your nervous system's response to stress.

Breathwork is a method of intentionally changing your breathing patterns in order to influence how you're feeling. When we are anxious or stressed (sympathetic system activation), we tend to take short, shallow breaths from the top part of our lungs by our chest. When we are relaxed (parasympathetic system activation), we tend to take longer, deeper breaths from the lower part of our lungs by our abdomen. In order to shift from a sympathetic state to a parasympathetic state, we can use breathwork practices to control our breath.

Pranayama (as used in yoga) is probably the most familiar breathwork practice, but there are many other types. The Art of Living is one organization that teaches breathwork practices and runs workshops around the world. There are many other options out there as well!

Breathwork may sound fancy or complicated, but it doesn't have to be. Sure, there are advanced breathwork practices for experienced practitioners. But even the simplest methods can give you a big bang for your buck. Breathwork offers a completely free, fairly fast, and highly effective intervention.

Play

Yes, if your mind went there, it could be sex. I would also suggest thinking more broadly. Infuse your life with fun— the real, old-fashioned kind. Sing, dance, laugh, imagine. Go on adventures. Create something new. The possibilities are endless. No holds barred. Get some freakin' fun in your life.

As you can see, there are many options for better approaching and managing stress. It's about having many tools in your toolkit so you have lots of techniques to choose from when stressful situations arise. Find what works for you, and forget the rest. If you change your relationship to stress, you will change how you experience your life. Don't run away from it. Acknowledge it, accept it, and work with it rather than against it.

CHAPTER SUMMARY

- You can measure how stressed your body is with specific lab tests.

- When the body is stressed, it diverts resources from making sex hormones to making stress hormones. This can have a profound effect on fertility.

- It is important to account for *both* psychological and physiological stressors when it comes to health and fertility.

- Chronic stress is more problematic for health than acute stress.

- To be better at stress, reframe how you think about it. Identify sources; then eliminate those that are unnecessary and manage what you can't eliminate.

- There are lots of tools to choose from to better manage stress, including meditation, tapping, gratitude, journaling, breathwork, and recreation. Experiment and see what resonates with you.

(16)

THE REAL SEX ED
Have Some Freakin' Fun!

STATUS CHECK

It's advisable to do one final health status check before you get the official trying-to-conceive (TTC) party started. Have you completed all follow-up items from your preconception visit (e.g., medication changes/tapering, immunizations)? Depending on what came up on your preconception lab work, you will likely want to rerun your preconception labs to ensure that any yellow or red flags have been addressed. You've done the legwork—let's confirm that everything looks good and you're ready to rock and roll!

You know you're physically ready to start trying to conceive when:

- Your pre-pregnancy wellness status is optimized across categories.

- Any chronic conditions are well managed.
- Any medications and supplements you're taking have been confirmed to be fertility and pregnancy safe.
- For females: Your hormones are balanced, your period is regular, and you've confirmed ovulation.
- You've optimized your environment and lifestyle to be as fertility friendly as possible.

If that's where you're at, then it's go time.

LET'S GET IT ON

Yes! You did it! You made it to the last chapter of the book. There has been a lot of planning and preparing that has occurred up to this point. Now it's finally time to discuss sex for conception. I'm technically getting ahead of myself here, since this is part of the "trying-to-conceive" phase, not the "preparing-to-conceive" phase, but what the heck? I know I've probably got a bunch of overachievers reading this, wanting to know it all right now.

Let's dive into a little modern-day sexual education. As we currently understand it, there is a six-day fertile window each month. Pregnancy can occur during this six-day fertile window, which includes the five days prior to ovulation as well as the day of ovulation itself.

The reason that the fertile window is six days long is twofold:

- Sperm can survive in a female's body for *up to five days*, though, on average, they tend to last closer to 1.5 days.

- An egg is only available for fertilization for up to twelve to twenty-four hours (and sometimes only six to twelve hours).

The "textbook" example is a woman with a twenty-eight-day cycle who ovulates on day fourteen, but each woman's cycle length is different. For this reason, it's important to know your cycle length and approximately when you are going to ovulate so that you can estimate your fertile window each month.

Once you know roughly when your fertile window is, when should you be having sex to optimize your chances of getting pregnant? There are certain days within your fertile window that are even more likely to yield a pregnancy. According to a seminal 1995 study, the most fertile days are one day and two days *prior* to ovulation and the day of ovulation itself. Here's why: the sperm needs to be *waiting* for the egg when it's released from the ovary. If you have sex after ovulation, it's likely too late to conceive that month.

Here is the nitty-gritty breakdown on the likelihood of conceiving by day of menstrual cycle:

- Six days before ovulation: 0 percent
- Five days before: 10 percent
- Four days before: 16 percent
- Three days before: 14 percent
- *Two days before: 27 percent*
- *One day before: 31 percent*
- *Day of ovulation: 33 percent*
- One day after ovulation: 0 percent[1]

Studies have varied on the optimal day for conception, but this is what the latest and greatest research tells us. Other studies suggest that one or two days before ovulation is the most fertile, but basically, it's the three-day window leading up to and including ovulation that's likely most fertile. It's probably a good bet to aim for at least one, if not all, of those three days.

Practically speaking, this means:

- Figure out when you're ovulating or when you're likely to ovulate.

- If you've been able to pinpoint approximately when you're ovulating, have sex the day before ovulation and the day of ovulation.

- If you're still not sure about when you're ovulating, consider having sex every other day for about a ten-day period prior to ovulation (e.g., from day eight to eighteen of your cycle if your cycle is twenty-six to thirty-two days long). Whoa, sexy time! This may be more frequent sex than usual for you, so be gentle with yourself and your partner as you navigate this process.

PUBLIC SERVICE ANNOUNCEMENT

Despite the entire section on ovulation tracking earlier in the book, I am going to say something that may seem contradictory. There is so much focus on timing sex for ovulation, and I think it's overkill. If you have a regular cycle, you can just aim to have sex several times mid-cycle, and you probably don't have to overthink it. For those with irregular cycles, I would encourage you to confirm that you are ovulating in the first place. If not, we have to troubleshoot that first.

Trying to conceive can be stressful. I have seen so many females drive themselves crazy trying to time sex—and driving their male partners crazy as a result. This stress can create pressure, expectations, and goal orientation. "On-demand" sex when you are ovulating puts a lot of pressure on you and your partner, and many people report trouble performing under pressure. Furthermore, stress can also dampen our libido and create distance from our partners. If sexual desire is the product of novelty and mystery, then baby-making sex is the exact antithesis of that—planned, routine, repetitive. It's the perfect storm of desire-killing characteristics. Many studies have confirmed this. Couples who are trying to have a baby report frequently that sex becomes like a chore, mechanical and routine.

The bottom line is that stress and sex don't mix. Figuring out how to get the stress out of your bedroom and the fun back into it is a key part of this journey. A bit of proactivity and creativity will go a long way in this department. Also, if there are things interfering with your enjoyment of sex (e.g., sexual pain, poor body image, unsaid things in your relationship), now would be the time to address them rather than waiting until you are actively trying to conceive. Believe me, I have seen this with many couples—trying to conceive brings everything to the surface. Might as well get in front of it now!

A BATTLE FOR THE AGES

Now that we've discussed ovulation, what happens next? Let's take a look at the epic journey that sperm take through the female body in pursuit of conception. This is how it goes down in a heterosexual couple who is conceiving naturally.

There are three main steps to getting pregnant: ejaculation, fertilization, and implantation.

Millions of sperm are created every day. Once created, each sperm ends up in a structure on top of the testes called the epididymis; they remain here until ejaculation. Once ejaculated, sperm have one goal—to deliver their genetic payload to the female egg.

Conception is the fiercest of competitions. On average, there are hundreds of millions of competitors at the outset. According to the documentary *The Great Sperm Race*, "The sperm will face death at every turn. There is no going back, no surrender, and only one winner."[2]

Within a few hours of entering the vagina, ~99 percent of sperm will be dead or dying.[3] Some sperm are not viable from the outset. Some are already dead; some hardly move at all or just twitch. Some have large heads. Some have small heads. Some have two heads.

For the sperm that are viable, they have to travel through an obstacle course designed to eliminate all but the best. On their way to the egg, the sperm must be deposited in the woman's vagina, make their way through the tiny opening of the cervix, swim all the way through the uterus, and finally reach the small doorway into the fallopian tubes. It is not an easy journey.

One of the reasons it takes millions of sperm cells to fertilize an egg is that when they arrive in the female body, they are bombarded by her immune system. Many sperm die instantly after they are released, destroyed by acidic fluids in the vagina. These acidic fluids are designed to kill anything that invades it. Since sperm are foreign cells, they are often considered an invading force, and as far as the female immune system is concerned, they need to be eliminated. Of the millions that start the journey, it is estimated that less than 1 percent make it to the cervix.[4] This is aided by the presence of fertile cervical mucus. For only a few brief hours each month, when an egg is released from an ovary during ovulation, the thick, sticky cervical mucus changes into a wet, slippery, and abundant stream that sperm can easily swim through.

The few and mighty sperm that have made it past the cervix now only have hours remaining to reach and fertilize the egg before they die. Once in the uterus, though, sperm are still under attack from the female immune system. In this case, immune cells attack and effectively destroy or inactivate sperm on their way to the fallopian tubes. This response is the body's way to prevent polyspermy, a condition wherein an egg is fertilized by more than one sperm. The long and harrowing journey helps ensure that only the best sperm get close to the egg.

Only a lucky few make it into the fallopian tubes. Sperm have to display the correct swimming characteristics and likely molecular signature to get through the juncture from the uterus to the fallopian tubes. However, the sperm that have made it this far are rewarded. The environment in the fallopian tubes is much more welcoming and accommodating than the vagina or the uterus; it has nutrients for sperm to nourish themselves, as well as optimal pH and ion concentration. Sperm can hang out here for hours or even days waiting for the egg.

Once the egg is ovulated, sperm have receptors to sense where the egg is and start moving toward it. The egg has a limited lifetime. Timing is everything—if sperm arrive too early or too late to meet the egg, they will perish.

At the site of fertilization, only a few sperm are left to fight for entry into the egg. At this point, sperm must first undergo several biochemical changes (called capacitation) to allow it to be able to penetrate the egg. Once capacitated, sperm die within a few hours, so there's no going back. Fertilization time is estimated at around twenty-four hours.

After capacitation, sperm are ready to fertilize the egg. To do so, they have to reach the nucleus of the egg, which is surrounded by a sticky, jelly-like coating. The sperm sprays enzymes from its head to dig through this sticky coating; the enzymes allow the sperm to dissolve a hole in the outer layer for entry. Through this hole, the sperm delivers its DNA into the egg. The membrane surrounding the egg is then instantly transformed into a rigid barrier so that no other sperm can enter. Fertilization has officially occurred!

However, just because fertilization has happened does not mean that pregnancy will ensue. Once the nucleus of the sperm is deposited inside the egg, a hybrid cell has been created, merging one cell from the biological mother and one from the biological father. The chromosomes of the egg and sperm will now match up to form the full chromosome array of the first cell of the new person, determining everything from sex to eye color. The information needed to determine the sex of a baby is stored in the sperm's head, which includes twenty-three chromosomes of DNA, including a gender chromosome (X chromosome for a female or Y chromosome for a male).

Now, the fertilized egg (called zygote) continues to move through the fallopian tube. The zygote travels through the fallopian tube to the uterus about three to five days after fertilization. The cell of the zygote continuously divides, eventually forming a blastocyst. The blastocyst stays in the uterus for several days before it implants in the endometrium, the inner lining of the uterine wall. This attachment process is called implantation. If the blastocyst does not implant in the endometrium, pregnancy will not occur. If implantation happens, the cells continue to divide, some developing into a baby and others forming the placenta. The placenta begins producing human chorionic gonadotropin (hCG), which can be found in a female's blood around eleven days after conception and slightly later in urine (hCG tests are what confirm pregnancy). Pregnancy has arrived!

According to Josleen Wilson, author of *The Pre-Pregnancy Planner*, "Scientists estimate that 15 percent of the time the ovum is incapable of being fertilized; and 25 percent of the time it is fertilized, then silently aborts. In addition, a certain number of ova never make it into the fallopian tube." Overall, it is estimated that a couple has an approximately 20 percent likelihood of conceiving in any given month.[5]

For a highly entertaining and helpful visual representation of this entire journey, I recommend checking out *The Great Sperm Race* documentary.

There you have it—the entire conception story! Now it's time for you to go make your own magic happen.

PRECONCEPTION TIP

If I leave you with one thing, let it be this: the better your sex, the better your chance of conception.

His pleasure matters. There aren't a ton of studies on this and many are done in fertility clinics with masturbation. However, the research has shown that the duration of sexual arousal is correlated with sperm concentration. In other words: the longer the pre-ejaculatory sexual arousal, the higher the sperm concentration.[6] Essentially, this suggests that the more turned on a man is, the more he will ejaculate.

Her pleasure matters. For women, better orgasms may also enhance fertility. While it isn't necessary for a woman to reach orgasm in order to conceive, some experts suggest that the intensity of the contractions that accompany an orgasm may help pull or carry sperm into the cervix and then the uterus. Basically, the idea is that orgasm contractions may facilitate sperm entry into the uterus. There are also suggestions that orgasm optimizes vaginal pH and ion concentration, which also contributes to conception. Again, this seems plausible but doesn't have much data to support it—yet. That being said, I think it's a valid enough hypothesis to include. It basically encourages you to orgasm more. Who's going to argue with me on that one?

It is also important to mention the obvious: the more you enjoy sex, the more likely you are to be having sex, so that's a factor at play here as well. Essentially, this section is to say that enjoyable sex is also the most fertility friendly. Consider this your permission slip to go have yourself lots of gourmet sex!

CHAPTER SUMMARY

- Each cycle, there is a six-day fertile window during which pregnancy can occur, which includes the five days prior to ovulation as well as the day of ovulation itself.

- If you have sex after ovulation, it's likely too late to conceive that month. Sperm needs to be waiting for the egg when it's released from the ovary.

- Having sex in the three-day window leading up to and including ovulation has the highest chance of conception.

- It is estimated that a couple has a ~15–25 percent likelihood of conceiving in any given month.

CONCLUSION

WHO ARE YOU BECOMING?

*"Transitions are important for us to pay
attention to. They provide enough of a gap in
our identity—we're in the process of changing
from who we were to who we're becoming—
to get us to pay attention to our inner life."*
—HALÉ SOFIA SCHATZ,
IF THE BUDDHA CAME TO DINNER

It is at times of transition like getting pregnant and becoming a parent that we can question where we've been and
where we are going. I want to share a few words of guidance
for the next stage. This is the chapter of paradoxes.

Having worked with hundreds of clients, I feel com-
pelled to make a few observations about the approaches
that seem to work well and those that work less well when
it comes to adopting new behaviors. Here are some tips for
the road ahead.

DITCH THE PERFECTIONISM

I just spent sixteen chapters telling you all the things that you can do to prepare in advance for pregnancy—all the things you can do to be in the best health possible to give your child the best foundation of health and happiness possible. Now I'm going to tell you to put things in perspective.

I've worked with so many clients trying to get pregnant. They are fierce. They are focused. They are dedicated. They are always analyzing, always calculating, always in their head. They are also incredibly hard on themselves: "I'm not doing enough. I'm not eating the 'right' diet or doing the exact 'right' things to get pregnant. I'm not the perfect bastion of health." They're well versed on the perils of eating non-organic food…and the potential negative health effects of gluten…and the threats of irradiated fish…and the toxins lurking in bathroom cabinets. *Lions and tigers and bears. Oh my!*

I am all for cleaning up your body and your environment whenever and however you can—I literally just wrote an entire book about it. But please, let's be reasonable. Don't let too much knowledge paralyze you. Don't overcomplicate things. Don't let the pursuit of health be yet another stressor. That defeats the purpose.

The goal here is not to make perfect health decisions 100 percent of the time; that's impractical and overwhelming. Aim to do a little bit better every day. Make small upgrades to your diet, your movement routine, or your stress management techniques every day, every week, every month. This is about doing better, not doing it all always. Eating organic most of the time wins you a gold star. If you find yourself stranded on a desert island with only non-organic apples available, it's going to be okay. Just breathe.

Sometimes, we have to get out of our head. Sometimes, we have to let go of the intense control. Sometimes, we have to do the best that we can in that moment, and that will have to be enough. The pursuit of perfectionism is exhausting. More to the point, it is incompatible with parenthood.

Perfectionism is the first thing that goes out the window when you become a parent. There is never a "perfect" time to get pregnant. There is no "perfect" way to do pregnancy. There is no "perfect" method of parenting, though some people may tell you otherwise. In fact, "perfect" and "parenting" probably shouldn't even be uttered in the same sentence. It's just not possible or desirable. You do the best that you can with the information and resources you have available to you at the time.

As it relates to pregnancy, get rid of your notions of the "perfect" timeline (i.e., you'll go off birth control today and then give yourself three months to normalize your cycles and then get pregnant within three months after that). Get rid of your notions of the "perfect" conception (i.e., it has to happen in this certain way). Get rid of your conceptions of the "perfect" birth (i.e., it has to be on the due date, it has to be a water birth).

Be intentional, not obsessive. Be progressing, not perfecting. Do your best. That's all you've got anyway.

You can't be both perfect and a parent. You have to pick one. Which do you choose?

LISTEN TO YOUR OWN INTUITION

This is where I tell you not to listen to what I just said. We tend to get very caught up in listening to external cues about our health. Health is a balance between internal cues (e.g., hunger, fatigue, pain) and external cues (e.g., lab test results, health articles, books—including this one!).

If you're too externally focused, you're not in tune with your body. It's time to take back control of your relationship to your body. You can certainly filter external information into your decision-making process, but when you completely cede control of your behavior over to "X" plan, you will feel out of control. Eventually, you will rebel in order to take back control.

If you want to be in control of your body, you must be in control of your choices. You are your own sort of expert—the expert on you. The expert on what feels right in your body. The expert on what works for you and what doesn't. The expert on what you are and are not willing to do. No one else can decide these things for you. Stop handing over your power to this eating plan or that exercise plan. Stop deferring to others on what is best for your body. Instead, tune in to your body, and make decisions from your internal knowledge. *Does this food make me feel energetic and vibrant when I eat it? Does this type of exercise feel good in my body? Does engaging in this health practice feel consistent with my goals and self-image?*

Take what's been shared in these chapters, see what resonates, and choose what works for you. Neither submission nor rebellion to health guidance is effective; integration is the key to optimal health.

RECOGNIZE THAT YOU CAN'T
DELEGATE YOUR HEALTH

At the end of the day, you are your own healer. Not your mother. Not your partner. Not your doctor. You are ultimately responsible for your own health and well-being. Only you can choose to be an engaged and active participant in your health management. Only you can educate yourself fully and completely. Only you can advocate for yourself. Most importantly, only you can take responsibility for yourself. You are the one that chooses what to eat, how to move, and who to be each and every day. Healthcare practitioners and wellness gurus can point you in the appropriate direction, but they can't do the work for you. That's all you.

Because here's the thing: health is the one thing that can't be delegated.

At home, you can delegate cleaning and chores and laundry. At work, you can delegate things you're not great at or things you're great at but don't enjoy. But you can't delegate exercise. You can't delegate sleep. You can't delegate meditation. You and you alone need to do these things. You have to make the commitment. You have to show up. You have to make it happen. Tom Bilyeu, founder of Quest Nutrition and Impact Theory, says it perfectly: the ultimate goal is "to be proud of yourself when you're by yourself."

You also can't delegate your health to your doctor, your acupuncturist, your masseuse, or your spiritual guru. They are mere guides on your journey. You alone need to walk the path, learn the lessons, and adjust course as needed. In order to make this possible, I'd suggest that you delegate *everywhere else* in your life so that you can free up the necessary time and mental space to make this happen. In life, there are few things that only you can do. Health is one of them. Make space for that to happen.

WHO ARE YOU BECOMING?

As our time together comes to a close, I want to take a step back from the nitty-gritty details of pre-pregnancy planning and remind us why we are doing this.

Some of the changes may feel overwhelming at times. You may wonder whether it really matters, whether it really makes a difference. The unfortunate reality is you won't know until it's too late. *Why not give it your best shot?*

As you are about to embark on this journey of becoming a parent, take advantage of this time to take a step back and reflect. Reflect on where you've been—what you're proud of and what you're less proud of, what you've stood for and what you've fallen for, what and whom you've prioritized, how much you've loved and laughed, how much you've given back, and how it all stacks up. Who have you been up until now? Do you like, admire, and respect that person?

As you look toward the future, ponder where you're going—what you want to focus on, what you want to build and who you want to build it with, how you want to be in the world and what you want to be known for, where you want to live and love, and how it all comes together. Who are you hoping to become? What kind of life do you want to design for yourself and your children?

Be intentional with your future. This entire book is about

not just letting the chips fall where they may but taking pro-active action toward the goals that you desire. This is just the beginning.

It's important to think about and define this now. Once you become a parent, there are so many excuses to lose your way—time constraints, money constraints, health constraints, etc., etc., etc. But it's precisely because you are a parent that you need to find and follow your own intentionally designed, uniquely crafted, and desire-led way. The more clarity you have on your desires, the quicker you can get to the job of being the best version of you. The more lit up you are in the world, the better spouse, parent, sibling, and community member you will be. And the better role model you will be for your children.

Remember, as Brené Brown says, "You can't give children what you don't have yourself. No matter how much importance you place on it."

Whether we like it or not, we are role models for our children. They will follow what we do, not necessarily what we say. If we leave clothes on the ground, they will too. If we eat quickly and voraciously, they will too. If we yell, they will too. Children learn predominantly by observation and experience, not just through words.

If you want to teach your children well, then train yourself well. They will pick up your habits—good, bad, or indifferent. At least make them worthwhile!

If you want to teach your children respect, respect yourself first. If you want to teach your children compassion, show yourself compassion first. If you want to teach your children patience, be patient with yourself first.

You can't teach your children something that you don't practice. You can't tell them not to eat candy if your car is full of candy wrappers. You can't tell them to play outside if they never see you playing outside (or moving your body). You can't tell them to sit down while eating if you're always eating on the run.

It's the oldest rule in the book, but we sometimes forget it: practice what you preach. If you aren't practicing it, you aren't really preaching it. Children will pick up on your disingenuousness. They will know you're not for real. They will know that they don't have to take it seriously either.

If you want your children to be healthy, choose health for yourself. If you want your children to be happy, choose happiness for yourself. Whatever you want to teach your children, embody it first. Otherwise, they will call BS. Otherwise, they will see through the act. Otherwise, you will be lying to yourself and lying to them.

Be the person you want your children to become. Maybe they follow suit; maybe they don't. You can't control that part. But at least you're in integrity, leading by example, and giving them the best possible shot you can.

You made it to the end of this book, which is really the beginning of your journey. Now it's time to start crafting the next chapter for yourself. Cheers!

APPENDICES

APPENDIX A: PRE-PREGNANCY WELLNESS TESTING

To access the most recent list of pre-pregnancy wellness testing biomarkers, please visit *www.getpoplin.com*. A quick overview of how to get pre-pregnancy wellness testing with Poplin in four steps:

1. **Order your test package online.** You can start your journey in less than five minutes by selecting one of Poplin's Pre-Pregnancy Wellness Tests.

2. **Get your labs done.** You can select to have your blood drawn at a local lab or in the comfort of your home with mobile phlebotomy. Either way, it's quick and efficient.

3. **View your personalized results.** Once your results are ready, you will receive a detailed report that outlines your pre-pregnancy wellness status. Each

biomarker result will include an explanation of what it is and why it is relevant for fertility and pregnancy.

4. **Schedule your educational call**. Once you have reviewed your test results, you can schedule a one-on-one educational call with our pre-pregnancy experts. This call will help you better understand your results and determine the best next steps for your pre-pregnancy journey.

APPENDIX B: RESOURCES

www.9monthsisnotenough.com/bookresources

NOTES

Introduction

1 Sara Gottfried, "Functional MD Support for How to Conceive Naturally," The Whole Journey, accessed March 31, 2023, https://www.thewholejourney.com/programs/fertility.

2 Catherine Shanahan and Luke Shanahan, *Deep Nutrition: Why Your Genes Need Traditional Food* (New York: Flatiron Books, 2017), 47.

3 Lee Warner et al., "Time for Public Health Action on Infertility," *Grand Rounds*, U.S. Centers for Disease Control and Prevention, presented on August 19, 2014, video, 1:10:29, https://www.cdc.gov/grand-rounds/pp/2014/20140819-infertility-pregnancy.html.

4 Committee on Gynecologic Practice, American Society for Reproductive Medicine, "ACOG Committee Opinion No. 762: Prepregnancy Counseling," *Obstetrics & Gynecology* 133, no. 1 (January 2019): e78–e89, https://doi.org/10.1097/AOG.0000000000003013.

1. Waiting to Address Fertility until It Becomes Infertility Is Way Too Late

1 "Is Infertility a Common Problem?" Infertility FAQS, Reproductive Health, U.S. Centers for Disease Control and Prevention, last modified March 10, 2023, https://www.cdc.gov/reproductivehealth/infertility/index.htm.

2 Sami David, "Maximum Fertility without IVF," DrSamiDavid.com, accessed March 31, 2023, http://www.drsamidavidmd.com/bio.

3 Lee Warner et al., "Time for Public Health Action on Infertility,"

298

Grand Rounds, U.S. Centers for Disease Control and Prevention, August 19, 2014, PowerPoint presentation, slide 16, https://stacks.cdc. gov/view/cdc/24794.

4   Alice D. Domar, Patricia C. Zuttermeister, and Richard Friedman, "The Psychological Impact of Infertility: A Comparison with Patients with Other Medical Conditions," *Journal of Psychosomatic Obstetrics and Gynaecology* 14 Suppl (1993): 45–52, https://pubmed.ncbi.nlm. nih.gov/8142988/.

5   "Money, Occupation and IVF Success Rates," FertilityIQ, accessed March 31, 2023, https://www.fertilityiq.com/topics/ivf/money-occupation-and-ivf-success-rates.

6   "ART Success Rates," Assisted Reproductive Technology (ART), U.S. Centers for Disease Control and Prevention, last modified February 21, 2023, https://www.cdc.gov/art/artdata/index.html#success.

7   "Costs of IVF," FertilityIQ, accessed March 31, 2023, https:// www.fertilityiq.com/ivf-in-vitro-fertilization/costs-of-ivf#cost-components.

8   "Modern State of Fertility 2020: Career & Money," Modern Fertility, Ro, accessed March 31, 2023, https://modernfertility.com/modern-state-fertility-2020-sofi-career-money.

9   Manuela Chiabvarini et al., "Cancer Risk in Children and Young Adults (Offspring) Born after Medically Assisted Reproduction: A Systematic Review and Meta-Analysis," *J* 2, no. 4 (October 2019): 430–448, https://doi.org/10.3390/j2040028; Liang Liu et al., "Association between Assisted Reproductive Technology and the Risk of Autism Spectrum Disorders in the Offspring: A Meta-Analysis," *Scientific Reports* 7 (April 2017): 46207, https://doi.org/10.1038/srep46207.

10 Ro, "Modern State of Fertility."

11 Christina D. Bethell et al., "A National and State Profile of Leading Health Problems and Health Care Quality for US Children: Key Insurance Disparities and Across-State Variations," *Academic Pediatrics* 11, no. 3 (May 2011): S22–S33, https://doi.org/10.1016/j. acap.2010.08.011.

2. Everything You've Been Told about Fertility Is Wrong

1   Henri Leridon, "Can Assisted Reproduction Technology Compensate for the Natural Decline in Fertility with Age? A Model Assessment," *Human Reproduction* 19, no. 7 (July 2004): 1548–1553, https://doi.org/10.1093/humrep/deh304.

2   David B. Dunson, Donna D. Baird, and Bernardo Colombo, "Increased Infertility with Age in Men and Women," *Obstetrics and Gynecology* 103, no. 1 (January 2004): 51–56, https://doi.org/10.1097/01.aog.0000100153.24061.45.

3   Luca Persani et al., "Primary Ovarian Insufficiency: X Chromosome Defects and Autoimmunity," *Journal of Autoimmunity* 33, no. 1 (August 2009): 35–41, https://doi.org/10.1016/j.jaut.2009.03.004; Omar Shebl et al., "Age-Related Distribution of Basal Serum AMH Level in Women of Reproductive Age and a Presumably Healthy Cohort," *Fertility and Sterility* 95, no. 2 (February 2011): 832–834, https://doi.org/10.1016/j.fertnstert.2010.09.012.

4   W. Hamish B. Wallace and Thomas W. Kelsey, "Human Ovarian Reserve from Conception to the Menopause," *PLoS One* 5, no. 1 (January 2010): e8772, https://doi.org/10.1371/journal.pone.0008772.

5   Rebecca Fett, *It Starts with the Egg: How the Science of Egg Quality Can Help You Get Pregnant Naturally, Prevent Miscarriage, and Improve Your Odds in IVF* (New York: Franklin Fox Publishing, 2016), 12.

6   Dan Buettner, "Power 9: Reverse Engineering Longevity," Blue Zones, accessed March 31, 2023, https://www.bluezones.com/2016/11/power-9/.

7   Sanjana Sood et al., "A Novel Multi-Tissue RNA Diagnostic of Healthy Ageing Relates to Cognitive Health Status," *Genome Biology* 16, no. 1 (2015): 185, https://doi.org/10.1186/s13059-015-0750-x.

8   WHO Scientific Group on Advances in Methods of Fertility, *Advances in Methods of Fertility Regulation*, World Health Organization Technical Report Series No. 575 (Geneva: World Health Organization, 1975), 11, https://apps.who.int/iris/bitstream/handle/10665/38635/WHO_TRS_575.pdf;jsessionid=67952FA4291A0DDADC5748677EACDA75?sequence=1.

9   Maura Palmery et al., "Oral Contraceptives and Changes in Nutritional Requirements," *European Review for Medical and Pharmacological Science* 17, no. 13 (July 2013): 1804–1813, https://pubmed.ncbi.nlm.nih.gov/23852908/.

10 Atousa Aminzadeh, Ali Sabeti Sanat, and Saeed Nik Akhtar, "Frequency of Candidiasis and Colonization of Candida albicans in Relation to Oral Contraceptive Pills," *Iran Red Crescent Medical Journal* 18, no. 10 (October 2016): e38909, https://doi.org/10.5812/ircmj.38909; Ronald Ortizo et al., "Exposure to Oral Contraceptives Increases the Risk for Development of Inflammatory Bowel Disease:

A Meta-Analysis of Case-Controlled and Cohort Studies," *European Journal of Gastroenterology and Hepatology* 29, no. 9 (September 2017): 1064–1070, https://doi.org/10.1097/meg.0000000000000915.

11 Noel T. Mueller et al., "The Infant Microbiome Development: Mom Matters," *Trends in Molecular Medicine* 21, no. 2 (February 2015): 109–117, https://doi.org/10.1016%2Fj.molmed.2014.12.002.

12 Rachel K. Jones, *Beyond Birth Control: The Overlooked Benefits of Oral Contraceptive Pills* (New York: Guttmacher Institute, 2011), 3, https://www.guttmacher.org/report/beyond-birth-control-overlooked-benefits-oral-contraceptive-pills.

13 F. Torre et al., "Effects of Oral Contraceptives on Thyroid Function and Vice Versa," *Journal of Endocrinological Investigation* 43, no. 9 (September 2020): 1181–1188, https://doi.org/10.1007/s40618-020-01230-8; Claudia Panzer et al., "Impact of Oral Contraceptives on Sex Hormone-Binding Globulin and Androgen Levels: A Retrospective Study in Women with Sexual Dysfunction," *The Journal of Sexual Medicine* 3, no. 1 (January 2006): 104–113, https://doi.org/10.1111/j.1743-6109.2005.00198.x; Marni A. Nenke et al., "Differential Effects of Estrogen on Corticosteroid-Binding Globulin Forms Suggests Reduced Cleavage in Pregnancy," *Journal of the Endocrine Society* 1, no. 3 (March 2017): 202–210, https://doi.org/10.1210/js.2016-1094.

14 Hagai Levine et al., "Temporal Trends in Sperm Count: A Systematic Review and Meta-Regression Analysis," *Human Reproduction Update* 23, no. 6 (November–December 2017): 646–659, https://doi.org/10.1093/humupd/dmx022.

15 "About Male Factor," Male Factor Infertility, RESOLVE: The National Infertility Association, accessed March 31, 2023, https://resolve.org/learn/infertility-101/underlying-causes/male-factor/.

16 Lynne Robinson et al., "The Effect of Sperm DNA Fragmentation on Miscarriage Rates: A Systematic Review and Meta-Analysis," *Human Reproduction* 27, no. 10 (October 2012): 2908–2917, https://doi.org/10.1093/humrep/des261.

17 Nicolás Garrido et al., "Sperm DNA Methylation Epimutation Biomarker for Paternal Offspring Autism Susceptibility," *Clinical Epigenetics* 13, no. 6 (2021): 1–13, https://doi.org/10.1186/s13148-020-00995-2.

18 Dunson, Baird, and Colombo, "Increased Infertility with Age," 51.

19 Dunson, Baird, and Colombo, "Increased Infertility with Age," 51.

20 Dunson, Baird, and Colombo, "Increased Infertility with Age," 51.

21 Sarah Druckenmiller Cascante et al., "Fifteen Years of Autologous Oocyte Thaw Outcomes from a Large University-Based Fertility Center," *Fertility and Sterility* 118, no. 1 (July 2022): 158–166, https://doi.org/10.1016/j.fertnstert.2022.04.013.

22 "ART Success Rates," Assisted Reproductive Technology (ART), U.S. Centers for Disease Control and Prevention, last modified February 21, 2023, https://www.cdc.gov/art/artdata/index.html#success.

23 "Money, Occupation and IVF Success Rates," FertilityIQ, accessed March 31, 2023, https://www.fertilityiq.com/topics/ivf/money-occupation-and-ivf-success-rates.

24 Yvonne A. R. White et al., "Oocyte Formation by Mitotically Active Germ Cells Purified from Ovaries of Reproductive-Age Women," *Nature Medicine* 18, no. 3 (March 2012): 413–421, https://doi.org/10.1038/nm.2669.

3. Why Getting Pregnant Is Harder Today
than for Previous Generations

1 Shanna Swan, *Count Down: How Our Modern World Is Threatening Sperm Counts, Altering Male and Female Reproductive Development, and Imperiling the Future of the Human Race* (New York: Scribner, 2020), 14.

2 Hagai Levine et al., "Temporal Trends in Sperm Count: A Systematic Review and Meta-Regression Analysis," *Human Reproduction Update* 23, no. 6 (November–December 2017): 646–659, https://doi.org/10.1093/humupd/dmx022.

3 *Food, Inc.*, directed by Robert Kenner (New York: Magnolia Pictures, 2009), 94 minutes, https://www.pbs.org/pov/films/foodinc/.

4 Jorge E. Chavarro et al., "Diet and Lifestyle in the Prevention of Ovulatory Disorder Infertility," *Obstetrics and Gynecology* 110, no. 5 (November 2007): 1050–1058, https://doi.org/10.1097/01.aog.0000287293.25465.e1; Elsje C. Oostingh et al., "Strong Adherence to a Healthy Dietary Pattern Is Associated with Better Semen Quality, Especially in Men with Poor Semen Quality," *Fertility and Sterility* 107, no. 4 (April 2017): 916–923, https://doi.org/10.1016/j.fertnstert.2017.02.103.

5 Jo Ellen Hinck et al., "Widespread Occurrence of Intersex in Black Basses (Micropterus spp.) from U.S. Rivers, 1995–2004," *Aquatic Toxicology* 95, no. 1 (October 2009): 60–70, https://doi.org/10.1016/j.aquatox.2009.08.001.

6   Adrianne P. Smits, David K. Skelly, and Susan R. Bolden, "Amphibian Intersex in Suburban Landscapes," *Ecosphere* 5, no. 1 (January 2014): 1–9, https://doi.org/10.1890/ES13-00353.1.

7   "About the TSCA Chemical Substance Inventory," TSCA Chemical Substance Inventory, United States Environmental Protection Agency, last modified June 29, 2022, https://www.epa.gov/tsca-inventory/about-tsca-chemical-substance-inventory.

8   Alisa L. Rich et al., "The Increasing Prevalence in Intersex Variation from Toxicological Dysregulation in Fetal Reproductive Tissue Differentiation and Development by Endocrine-Disrupting Chemicals," *Environmental Health Insights* 10 (January–February 2016): 163–171, https://doi.org/10.4137/EHI.S39825.

9   Sheldon Cohen and Denise Janicki-Deverts, "Who's Stressed? Distributions of Psychological Stress in the United States in Probability Samples from 1983, 2006, and 2009," *Journal of Applied Social Psychology* 42, no. 6 (June 2012): 1320–1334, https://doi.org/10.1111/j.1559-1816.2012.00900.x.

10 Joanna Jurewicz et al., "Wpływ stresu aawodowego na jakość nasienia," [The effect of stress on the semen quality], *Medycyna Pracy* 61, no. 6 (2010): 607–613, https://pubmed.ncbi.nlm.nih.gov/21452563/.

11 Giulia Collodel et al., "Effect of Emotional Stress on Sperm Quality," *Indian Journal of Medical Research* 128, no. 3 (September 2008): 254–261, https://pubmed.ncbi.nlm.nih.gov/19052335/.

12 "The Staggering Effects of Physical Inactivity," *The Pulse* (blog), You're the Cure, American Heart Association, July 23, 2013, https://www.yourethecure.org/the-staggering-effects-of-physical-inactivity.

13 Deborah Rohm Young et al., "Sedentary Behavior and Cardiovascular Morbidity and Mortality: A Science Advisory from the American Heart Association," *Circulation* 134, no. 13 (September 27, 2016): e262–e279, https://doi.org/10.1161/CIR.0000000000000440; Emily N. Ussery et al., "Joint Prevalence of Sitting Time and Leisure-Time Physical Activity among US Adults, 2015–2016," *The Journal of the American Medical Association* 320, no. 19 (2018): 2036–2038, https://doi.org/10.1001/jama.2018.17797.

14 Gwendoline de Fleurian et al., "Occupational Exposures Obtained by Questionnaire in Clinical Practice and Their Association with Semen Quality," *Journal of Andrology* 30, no. 5 (September–October 2009): 566–579, https://doi.org/10.2164/jandrol.108.005918.

15   Miguel Ángel Rosety et al., "Exercise Improved Semen Quality
     and Reproductive Hormone Levels in Sedentary Obese Adults,"
     Nutrición Hospitalaria 34, no. 3 (May–June 2017): 608–612, http://
     dx.doi.org/10.20960/nh.549.
16   M. Rosety-Rodriguez et al., "El entrenamiento en tapiz rodante
     a domicilio mejora la calidad seminal en adultos con diabetes
     de tipo 2," [Home-based treadmill training improved seminal
     quality in adults with type 2 diabetes], *Actas Urológicas Españolas*
     38, no. 9 (November 2014): 589–593, https://doi.org/10.1016/j.
     acuro.2013.10.013.
17   E. V. Bräuner et al., "The Association between In-Utero Exposure
     to Stressful Life Events during Pregnancy and Male Reproductive
     Function in a Cohort of 20-Year-Old Offspring: The Raine Study,"
     Human Reproduction 34, no. 7 (July 2019): 1345–1355, https://doi.
     org/10.1093/humrep/dez070; E. V. Bräuner et al., "The Association
     between In-Utero Exposure to Maternal Psychological Stress and
     Female Reproductive Function in Adolescence: A Prospective
     Cohort Study," *Comprehensive Psychoneuroendocrinology*
     5 (February 2021): 100026, https://doi.org/10.1016/j.
     cpnec.2020.100026.

Part 2. The Solution

1   "Planning for Pregnancy," Before Pregnancy, U.S. Centers for
     Disease Control and Prevention, last modified February 15, 2023,
     https://www.cdc.gov/preconception/planning.html.

4. Start Preparing Earlier

1   Preconception Health, *The Lancet*, April 17, 2018, https://www.
     thelancet.com/series/preconception-health.

5. Build Generational Health

1   Atul Malhotra et al., "Neonatal Morbidities of Fetal Growth
     Restriction: Pathophysiology and Impact," *Frontiers
     in Endocrinology* 10 (2019): 55, https://doi.org/10.3389/
     fendo.2019.00055.
2   Yong Hee Hong and Ji-Eun Lee, "Large for Gestational Age and
     Obesity-Related Comorbidities," *Journal of Obesity and Metabolic
     Syndrome* 30, no. 2 (2021): 124–131, https://doi.org/10.7570/jomes20130.

3   Judith Stephenson et al., "Preconception Health in England: A Proposal for Annual Reporting with Core Metrics," *The Lancet* 393, no. 10187 (June 2019): 2262–2271, https://doi.org/10.1016/S0140-6736(19)30954-7.

4   Maud Fagny et al., "The Epigenomic Landscape of African Rainforest Hunter-Gatherers and Farmers," *Nature Communications* 6 (2015): 10047, https://doi.org/10.1038/ncomms10047.

5   Hilary Parker, "A Moment with…Eric Lander '78," *Princeton Alumni Weekly*, January 28, 2009, https://paw.princeton.edu/article/moment-eric-lander-78.

6   "Epigenomics Fact Sheet," National Human Genome Research Institute, last modified August 16, 2020, https://www.genome.gov/about-genomics/fact-sheets/Epigenomics-Fact-Sheet.

7   Giuseppe Passarino, Francesco De Rango, and Alberto Montesanto, "Human Longevity: Genetics or Lifestyle? It Takes Two to Tango," *Immunity and Ageing* 13 (2016): 12, https://doi.org/10.1186/s12979-016-0066-z.

8   Shanna Swan, *Count Down: How Our Modern World Is Threatening Sperm Counts, Altering Male and Female Reproductive Development, and Imperiling the Future of the Human Race* (New York: Scribner, 2020), 133.

9   Mark Hyman, "The Failure of Decoding the Human Genome and the Future of Medicine," *Dr. Hyman* (blog), accessed March 31, 2023, https://drhyman.com/blog/2010/12/31/the-failure-of-decoding-the-human-genome-and-the-future-of-medicine/.

10 Ling Wu et al., "Paternal Psychological Stress Reprograms Hepatic Gluconeogenesis in Offspring," *Cell Metabolism* 23, no. 4 (April 2016): 735–743, https://doi.org/10.1016/j.cmet.2016.01.014; University of Southampton, "Risk of Obesity Influenced by Changes in Our Genes," news release, April 26, 2017, ScienceDaily, https://www.sciencedaily.com/releases/2017/04/170426093316.htm; Karen A. Lillycrop et al., "Association between Perinatal Methylation of the Neuronal Differentiation Regulator HES1 and Later Childhood Neurocognitive Function and Behaviour," *International Journal of Epidemiology* 44, no. 4 (August 2015): 1263–1276, https://doi.org/10.1093/ije/dyv052; Ali B. Rodgers et al., "Transgenerational Epigenetic Programming via Sperm MicroRNA Recapitulates Effects of Paternal Stress," *Proceedings of the National Academy of Sciences of the United States of America* 112, no. 44 (November 2015): 13699–13704, https://doi.org/10.1073/pnas.1508347112; Mariana

Schroeder et al., "A Methyl-Balanced Diet Prevents CRF-Induced Prenatal Stress-Triggered Predisposition to Binge Eating-Like Phenotype," *Cell Metabolism* 25, no. 6 (June 2017): 1269–1281, https://doi.org/10.1016/j.cmet.2017.05.001.

11 Swan, *Count Down*, 129.

12 Suneeta Senapati, "Infertility: A Marker of Future Health Risk in Women?" *Fertility and Sterility* 110, no. 5 (October 2018): 783–789, https://doi.org/10.1016/j.fertnstert.2018.08.058.

13 Swan, *Count Down*, 129–132.

6. Is Your Body Baby-Ready?

1 "Section 9: Natural History and Spectrum Disease," Lesson 1: Introduction to Epidemiology, U.S. Centers for Disease Control and Prevention, last modified May 18, 2012, https://www.cdc.gov/csels/dsepd/ss1978/lesson1/section9.html.

2 U.S. Centers for Disease Control and Prevention, "Section 9."

3 "Anemia during Pregnancy," American Pregnancy Association, accessed March 31, 2023, https://americanpregnancy.org/healthy-pregnancy/pregnancy-concerns/anemia-during-pregnancy/.

4 "Pelvic Inflammatory Disease (PID)—CDC Detailed Fact Sheet," Facts and Brochures, Pelvic Inflammatory Disease (PID), Sexually Transmitted Diseases (STDs), U.S. Centers for Disease Control and Prevention, last modified July 22, 2021, https://www.cdc.gov/std/pid/stdfact-pid-detailed.htm.

5 "Perinatal Transmission," Hepatitis B Information, Viral Hepatitis, U.S. Centers for Disease Control and Prevention, last modified February 16, 2022, https://www.cdc.gov/hepatitis/hbv/perinatalxmtn.htm; "Prevent Perinatal Transmission," Prevention, HIV Basics, HIV, U.S. Centers for Disease Control and Prevention, last modified February 2, 2023, https://www.cdc.gov/hiv/basics/hiv-prevention/mother-to-child.html.

6 Maunil K. Desai and Roberta Diaz Brinton, "Autoimmune Disease in Women: Endocrine Transition and Risk across the Lifespan," *Frontiers in Endocrinology* 10 (2019): 265, https://doi.org/10.3389/fendo.2019.00265.

7 Paul P. Doghramji, *Screening and Laboratory Diagnosis of Autoimmune Diseases Using Antinuclear Antibody Immunofluorescence Assay and Specific Autoantibody Testing*, MI6203 (Secaucus, NJ: Quest Diagnostics, 2016), 2, https://www.

aafp.org/dam/AAFP/documents/about_us/sponsored_resources/ Quest_%20ANA-IFA_Monograph.pdf.

8   Ricard Cervera and Juan Balasch, "Autoimmunity and Recurrent Pregnancy Losses," *Clinical Reviews in Allergy & Immunology* 39, no. 3 (2010): 148–152, https://doi.org/10.1007/s12016-009-8179-1.

9   Doghramji, *Screening and Laboratory Diagnosis*, 6.

10 Spyridoula Maraka et al., "Subclinical Hypothyroidism in Women Planning Conception and during Pregnancy: Who Should Be Treated and How?" *Journal of the Endocrine Society* 2, no. 6 (June 2018): 533–546, https://doi.org/10.1210/js.2018-00090.

11 Tetsurou Sakumoto et al., "Insulin Resistance/Hyperinsulinemia and Reproductive Disorders in Infertile Women," *Reproductive Medicine and Biology* 9, no. 4 (December 2010): 185–190, https://doi.org/10.1007/s12522-010-0062-5.

12 Änne Bartels and Keelin O'Donoghue, "Cholesterol in Pregnancy: A Review of Knowns and Unknowns," *Obstetric Medicine* 4, no. 4 (2011): 147–151, https://doi.org/10.1258/om.2011.110003.

13 Folami Y. Ideraabdullah et al., "Maternal Vitamin D Deficiency and Developmental Origins of Health and Disease (DOHaD)," *Journal of Endocrinology* 241, no. 2 (2019): R65–R80, https://doi.org/10.1530/JOE-18-0541.

14 "Guide to Sperm Quality," Legacy, accessed March 31, 2023, https://www.givelegacy.com/sperm-quality/.

7. To Screen or Not to Screen?

1   "Considering Having a Baby? Carrier Screening Is for You," Invitae, accessed March 31, 2023, https://www.invitae.com/en/pregnancy/carrier-screen.

2   "ACOG Recommends Offering Additional Carrier Screening to All Women, Regardless of Ethnicity or Family History," news release, February 27, 2017, Clinical, American College of Obstetricians and Gynecologists, https://www.acog.org/news/news-releases/2017/02/acog-recommends-offering-additional-carrier-screening-to-all-women.

3   Committee on Genetics, American College of Obstetricians and Gynecologists, "Committee Opinion No. 690: Carrier Screening in the Age of Genomic Medicine," *Obstetrics and Gynecology* 129, no. 3 (March 2017): e36, https://doi.org/10.1097/AOG.0000000000001947.

4   Committee on Genetics, "Opinion No. 690," e37.

5   Fred Levine, "Chapter 1: Basic Genetic Principals," in *Fetal and Neonatal Physiology: Volume 1*, 3rd ed., eds. Richard A. Polin, William W. Fox, and Steven H. Abman (Philadelphia: W. B. Saunders, 2004): 1–15, https://doi.org/10.1016/B978-0-7216-9654-6.50004-7.

8. *The Most Impactful Doctor's Visit of Your Life*

1   Committee on Gynecologic Practice, American College of Obstetricians and Gynecologists, and American Society for Reproductive Medicine, "Committee Opinion No. 762: Prepregnancy Counseling," *Obstetrics and Gynecology* 133, no. 1 (January 2019): e78–e89, https://doi.org/10.1097/AOG.0000000000003013; "Preconception Health and Health Care Is Important for All," Before Pregnancy, U.S. Centers for Disease Control and Prevention, last modified January 11, 2023, https://www.cdc.gov/preconception/overview.html.

2   Kay Johnson et al., "Recommendations to Improve Preconception Health and Health Care—United States: A Report of the CDC/ATSDR Preconception Care Work Group and the Select Panel on Preconception Care," *Morbidity and Mortality Weekly Report* 55, no. RR06 (April 21, 2006): 1–23, https://www.cdc.gov/mmwr/preview/mmwrhtml/rr5506a1.htm.

3   Cheryl L. Robbins et al., "Core State Preconception Health Indicators—Pregnancy Risk Assessment Monitoring System and Behavioral Risk Factor Surveillance System, 2009," *Morbidity and Mortality Weekly Report* 63, no. SS03 (April 25, 2014): 7, https://www.cdc.gov/mmwr/preview/mmwrhtml/ss6303a1.htm.

4   "Preconception Health and Health Care," U.S. Centers for Disease Control and Prevention, accessed March 31, 2023, http://medbox.iiab.me/modules/en-cdc/www.cdc.gov/preconception/overview.html.

5   Johnson et al., "Recommendations to Improve Preconception Health," 2.

6   Christine Dehlendorf et al., "Evolving the Preconception Health Framework," *Obstetrics and Gynecology* 137, no. 2 (February 2021): 235, https://doi.org/10.1097/AOG.0000000000004255.

7   American Diabetes Association, "Management of Diabetes in Pregnancy: Standards of Medical Care in Diabetes—2021," *Diabetes Care* 44, no. Supplement_1 (January 2021): S200–S210, https://doi.org/10.2337/dc21-S014.

8   Jeffrey R. Garber et al., "Clinical Practice Guidelines for
    Hypothyroidism in Adults," *Endocrine Practice* 18, no. 6 (November
    2012): 988–1028, https://doi.org/10.4158/EP12280.GL.

9   U.S. Department of Health and Human Services, "Chapter
    9: Reproductive Outcomes," in *The Health Consequences of
    Smoking—50 Years of Progress: A Report of the Surgeon General*
    (Atlanta: U.S. Centers for Disease Control and Prevention, 2014),
    459–522, https://www.ncbi.nlm.nih.gov/books/NBK294307/.

10 Madeline F. Perry, Helen Mulcahy, and Emily A. DeFranco,
    "Influence of Periconception Smoking Behavior on Birth
    Defect Risk," *American Journal of Obstetrics and Gynecology*
    220, no. 6 (June 2019): 558.E1–588.E7, https://doi.org/10.1016/j.
    ajog.2019.02.029.

11 Johnson et al., "Recommendations to Improve Preconception
    Health," 5.

12 Roger Hart et al., "Periodontal Disease: A Potential Modifiable Risk
    Factor Limiting Conception," *Human Reproduction* 27, no. 5 (May
    2012): 1332–1342, https://doi.org/10.1093/humrep/des034.

13 Ben-Juan Wei et al., "Periodontal Disease and Risk of
    Preeclampsia: A Meta-Analysis of Observational Studies," *PLoS
    One* 8, no. 8 (2013): e70901, https://doi.org/10.1371/journal.
    pone.0070901; Rajiv Saini, Santosh Saini, and Sugandha R. Saini,
    "Periodontitis: A Risk for Delivery of Premature Labor and Low-
    Birth-Weight Infants," *Journal of Natural Science, Biology, and
    Medicine* 1, no. 1 (July 2010): 40–42, https://www.ncbi.nlm.nih.
    gov/pmc/articles/PMC3217279/.

14 Nicole A. Huijgen et al., "Are Proton-Pump Inhibitors Harmful
    for the Semen Quality of Men in Couples Who Are Planning
    Pregnancy?" *Fertility and Sterility* 106, no. 7 (December 2016):
    1666–1672, https://doi.org/10.1016/j.fertnstert.2016.09.010; Jiarong
    Xu et al., "The Effect of SSRIs on Semen Quality: A Systematic
    Review and Meta-Analysis," *Frontiers in Pharmacology* 13 (2022):
    911489, https://doi.org/10.3389/fphar.2022.911489.

9. It's Not You; It's Your Environment

1   David L. Katz, *Disease Proof: The Remarkable Truth about What
    Makes Us Well* (New York: Hudson Street Press, 2013), xv.

2   Monica K. Silver and John D. Meeker, "Chapter 13: Endocrine
    Disruption of Developmental Pathways and Children's Health," in

Endocrine Disruption and Human Health, ed. Philippa D. Darbre (Cambridge, MA: Academic Press, 2015), 237–255, https://doi.org/10.1016/B978-0-12-801139-3.00013-2.

3   "Planning for Pregnancy," Before Pregnancy, U.S. Centers for Disease Control and Prevention, last modified February 15, 2023, https://www.cdc.gov/preconception/planning.html.

4   Environmental Working Group, *Pollution in People: Cord Blood Contaminants in Minority Newborns* (Washington, D.C.: Environmental Working Group, 2009), 3, https://static.ewg.org/reports/2009/minority_cord_blood/2009-Minority-Cord-Blood-Report.pdf?_gl=1*1ay2mxh*_ga*OTE2OTM4NTUuMTY4MDYxNTAwNQ..*_ga_CS21GC49KT*MTY4MDYxNTAwNS4xLjEuMTY4MDYxNTAoNS4wLjAuMA.

5   "About the TSCA Chemical Substance Inventory," TSCA Chemical Substance Inventory, United States Environmental Protection Agency, last modified June 29, 2022, https://www.epa.gov/tsca-inventory/about-tsca-chemical-substance-inventory; *Food, Inc.*, directed by Robert Kenner (New York: Magnolia Pictures, 2009), 94 minutes, https://www.pbs.org/pov/films/foodinc/.

6   Daniel Ruiz and Heather Patisaul, eds., "Endocrine-Disrupting Chemicals (EDCs)," Patient Resources, Endocrine Society, January 24, 2022, https://www.endocrine.org/patient-engagement/endocrine-library/edcs.

7   Andrea C. Gore et al., *Introduction to Endocrine Disrupting Chemicals (EDCs): A Guide for Public Interest Organizations and Policy-Makers* (Washington, D.C.: Endocrine Society, December 2014), 1, https://www.endocrine.org/-/media/endosociety/files/advocacy-and-outreach/important-documents/introduction-to-endocrine-disrupting-chemicals.pdf.

8   Gore et al., *Introduction to EDCs*, 20.

9   Gore et al., *Introduction to EDCs*, 27.

10 Keerthi Priya et al., "Implications of Environmental Toxicants on Ovarian Follicles: How It Can Adversely Affect the Female Fertility?" *Environmental Science and Pollution Research* 28, no. 48 (2021): 67925–67939, https://doi.org/10.1007/s11356-021-16489-4.

11 Gore et al., *Introduction to EDCs*, 20.

12 Priya et al., "Implications of Environmental Toxicants," 67932–67933.

13 Aditi Sharma et al., "Endocrine-Disrupting Chemicals and Male Reproductive Health," *Reproductive Medicine and Biology* 19, no. 3 (July 2020): 243–253, https://doi.org/10.1002/rmb2.12326.

14 Gore et al., *Introduction to EDCs*, 20–21, 27, 45.

15 "How Reproductive Hazards Can Affect Your Health," Women's Fertility and Menstrual Function, Reproductive Health and the Workplace, Workplace Safety and Health Topics, National Institute for Occupational Safety and Health (NIOSH), U.S. Centers for Disease Control and Prevention, last modified April 20, 2017, https://www.cdc.gov/niosh/topics/repro/femaleHealthImpact.html.

16 Priya et al., "Implications of Environmental Toxicants," 67933–67934; Sharma et al., "EDCs and Male Reproductive Health," 245–246.

17 U.S. Centers for Disease Control and Prevention, "How Reproductive Hazards."

18 Neil E. Klepeis et al., "The National Human Activity Pattern Survey (NHAPS): A Resource for Assessing Exposure to Environmental Pollutants," *Journal of Exposure Science and Environmental Epidemiology* 11, no. 3 (2001): 231–252, https://doi.org/10.1038/sj.jea.7500165.

19 "Why Indoor Air Quality Is Important to Schools," United States Environmental Protection Agency, last modified December 5, 2022, https://www.epa.gov/iaq-schools/why-indoor-air-quality-important-schools.

20 American Society of Heating, Refrigerating and Air-Conditioning Engineers, *2016 ASHRAE Handbook—HVAC Systems and Equipment* (Peachtree Corners, GA: ASHRAE, 2016), 22.1, https://www.ashrae.org/file%20library/technical%20resources/covid-19/i-p_s16_ch22humidifiers.pdf.

21 Rockaway Borough Water Department, *Year 2021 Annual Water Quality Report*, PWSID#: NJ1434001 (Rockaway, NJ: Rockaway Borough Water Department, 2022), 1, https://www.rockawayborough.org/departments/publicworks/WaterQualityReport2021.pdf.

22 Rockaway Borough Water Department, *Water Quality Report*, 1.

23 "Exposures Add Up—Survey Results," Environmental Working Group, December 15, 2004, https://www.ewg.org/news-insights/news/2004/12/exposures-add-survey-results#.WYIpyoTyvZY.

24 "FDA Authority over Cosmetics: How Cosmetics Are Not FDA-Approved, but Are FDA-Regulated," Cosmetics Laws and Regulations, Cosmetics Guidance and Regulation, Cosmetics, U.S. Food and Drug Administration, last modified March 2, 2022, https://www.fda.gov/cosmetics/cosmetics-laws-regulations/fda-

authority-over-cosmetics-how-cosmetics-are-not-fda-approved-are-
fda-regulated.
25 Federal Food, Drug, and Cosmetic Act, 21 U.S.C. §§ 321–399i (1938).
26 "Cosmetic Products Regulation, Annex II—Prohibited Substances,"
European Chemicals Agency, last modified April 4, 2023, https://
echa.europa.eu/cosmetics-prohibited-substances; "Cosmetic
Ingredient Hotlist," Health Canada, Government of Canada, last
modified August 26, 2022, https://www.canada.ca/en/health-
canada/services/consumer-product-safety/cosmetics/cosmetic-
ingredient-hotlist-prohibited-restricted-ingredients/hotlist.html.
27 "Prohibited and Restricted Ingredients in Cosmetics," Cosmetics
Laws and Regulations, Cosmetics Guidance and Regulation,
Cosmetics, U.S. Food and Drug Administration, last modified
February 25, 2022, https://www.fda.gov/cosmetics/cosmetics-laws-
regulations/prohibited-restricted-ingredients-cosmetics; Office
of the Press Secretary, "Statement by the Press Secretary on H.R.
1321, S. 2425," Statements and Releases, Briefing Room, The White
House of President Barack Obama, December 28, 2015, https://
obamawhitehouse.archives.gov/the-press-office/2015/12/28/
statement-press-secretary-hr-1321-s-2425; U.S. Food and Drug
Administration, "FDA Issues Final Rule on Safety and Effectiveness
of Antibacterial Soaps," FDA news release, September 2, 2016,
https://www.fda.gov/news-events/press-announcements/fda-issues-
final-rule-safety-and-effectiveness-antibacterial-soaps.
28 https://www.ewg.org/skindeep/?gclid=EAIaIQobChMI8cKMrMK
51QIV20KzCh1JIw5iEAAYASABEgJsu_D_BwE#.WYJHYYTyvZY.
29 Kavindra Kumar Kesari, Ashok Agarwal, and Ralf Henkel,
"Radiations and Male Fertility," Reproductive Biology and
Endocrinology 16 (2018): 118, https://doi.org/10.1186/s12958-018-
0431-1.
30 Ariel Zilberlicht et al., "Habits of Cell Phone Usage and Sperm
Quality—Does It Warrant Attention?" Reproductive Biomedicine
Online 31, no. 3 (September 2015): 421–426, https://doi.org/10.1016/j.
rbmo.2015.06.006.
31 Mehmet Erol Yildirim et al., "What Is Harmful for Male Fertility:
Cell Phone or the Wireless Internet?" Kaohsiung Journal of
Medical Sciences 31, no. 9 (September 2015): 480–484, https://doi.
org/10.1016/j.kjms.2015.06.006.
32 Carly Hyland et al., "Organic Diet Intervention Significantly
Reduces Urinary Pesticide Levels in U.S. Children and Adults,"

Environmental Research 171 (April 2019): 568–575, https://doi. org/10.1016/j.envres.2019.01.024.

10. The Fertile Zone

1   We can also calculate Free Androgen Index, which can be an indicator of polycystic ovary syndrome (PCOS) from testosterone and SHBG levels.

2   "Weight," American Society for Reproductive Medicine, accessed March 31, 2023, https://www.asrm.org/topics/topics-index/weight/.

3   Natalia Hetemäki et al., "Adipose Tissue Estrogen Production and Metabolism in Premenopausal Women," *The Journal of Steroid Biochemistry and Molecular Biology* 209 (May 2021): 105849, https:// doi.org/10.1016/j.jsbmb.2021.105849.

4   Meaghan A. Leddy, Michael L. Power, and Jay Schulkin, "'The Impact of Maternal Obesity on Maternal and Fetal Health," *Reviews in Obstetrics and Gynecology* 1, no. 4 (Fall 2008): 170–178, https:// pubmed.ncbi.nlm.nih.gov/19173021/.

5   Zhen Han et al., "Maternal Underweight and the Risk of Preterm Birth and Low Birth Weight: A Systematic Review and Meta-Analyses," *International Journal of Epidemiology* 40, no. 1 (February 2011): 65–101, https://doi.org/10.1093/ije/dyq195.

6   Henrikki Nordman, Jarmo Jääskeläinen, and Raimo Voutilainen, "Birth Size as a Determinant of Cardiometabolic Risk Factors in Children," *Hormone Research in Paediatrics* 93, no. 3 (September 2020): 144–153, https://doi.org/10.1159/000509932.

7   Judith Brown, *Nutrition through the Life Cycle*, 7th ed. (Boston: Cengage, 2020), 95–96.

8   Dan Guo et al., "The Impact of BMI on Sperm Parameters and the Metabolite Changes of Seminal Plasma Concomitantly," *Oncotarget* 8, no. 30 (2017): 48619–48634, https://doi.org/10.18632/ oncotarget.14950.

9   E. M. Luque et al., "Body Mass Index and Human Sperm Quality: Neither One Extreme nor the Other," *Reproduction, Fertility and Development* 29, no. 4 (2015): 731–739, https://doi.org/10.1071/ rd15351.

10   Min-Ji Kim et al., "Fate and Complex Pathogenic Effects of Dioxins and Polychlorinated Biphenyls in Obese Subjects before and after Drastic Weight Loss," *Environmental Health Perspectives* 119, no. 3 (March 2011): 377–383, https://doi.org/10.1289/ehp.1002848.

11. The Foundation of Fertility

1 Note: one regular pad or tampon = 5 mL, one super pad/tampon = 10 mL.

2 A few caveats here: Blood is lighter when it's flowing quickly (e.g., at beginning /middle of period) and darker when it's flowing slowly (e.g., at end of period). Blood turns darker when it's exposed to air (such as on a sanitary pad over time), usually to a dark red/maroon or brown color. Very dark red or brown period blood can often appear at the beginning or end of your cycle; this is normal. It is when these colors appear regularly throughout your cycle that it may become a cause for further exploration.

3 Jolene Brighten, *Beyond the Pill: A 30-Day Program to Balance Your Hormones, Reclaim Your Body, and Reverse the Dangerous Side Effects of the Birth Control Pill* (New York: HarperOne, 2019).

4 Brighten, *Beyond the Pill*.

5 Sarah Johnson, Lorrae Marriott, and Michael Zinaman, "Can Apps and Calendar Methods Predict Ovulation with Accuracy?" *Current Medical Research and Opinion* 34, no. 9 (2018): 1587–1594, https://doi.org/10.1080/03007995.2018.1475348.

12. Eat as If You're Already Pregnant

1 Mary Barker et al., "Intervention Strategies to Improve Nutrition and Health Behaviours before Conception," *The Lancet* 391, no. 10132 (May 2018): 1853–1864, https://doi.org/10.1016/S0140-6736(18)30313-1.

2 "Folic Acid: The Best Tool to Prevent Neural Tube Defects," Articles and Key Findings, Folic Acid, U.S. Centers for Disease Control and Prevention, last modified September 9, 2022, https://www.cdc.gov/ncbddd/folicacid/features/folic-acid-helps-prevent-some-birth-defects.html.

3 Christopher S. Kovacs, "Bone Development and Mineral Homeostasis in the Fetus and Neonate: Roles of the Calciotropic and Phosphotropic Hormones," *Physiological Reviews* 94, no. 4 (October 2014): 1143–1218, https://doi.org/10.1152/physrev.00014.2014.

4 Jorge E. Chavarro et al., "Diet and Lifestyle in the Prevention of Ovulatory Disorder Infertility," *Obstetrics and Gynecology* 110, no. 5 (November 2007): 1050–1058, https://doi.org/10.1097/01.aog.0000287293.25465.e1.

5 Hillary Wright, "Fertility Diet Advice," Boston IVF Wellness Center, accessed March 31, 2023, https://www.bostonivf.com/wellness-center/fertility-diet-advice/.

6 Nim Barnes, *How to Conceive Healthy Babies the Natural Way* (London: New Generation Publishing, 2014).

7 As of 2022: strawberries, spinach, kale/collard/mustard greens, nectarines, apples, grapes, bell and hot peppers, cherries, peaches, pears, celery, and tomatoes. See For full details, see: https://www.ewg.org/foodnews/dirty-dozen.php for full details.

8 Marcin Barański et al., "Higher Antioxidant and Lower Cadmium Concentrations and Lower Incidence of Pesticide Residues in Organically Grown Crops: A Systematic Literature Review and Meta-Analyses," *British Journal of Nutrition* 112, no. 5 (2014): 794–811, https://doi.org/10.1017/s0007114514001366.

9 Dominika Średnicka-Tober et al., "Higher PUFA and N-3 PUFA, Conjugated Linoleic Acid, α-Tocopherol and Iron, But Lower Iodine and Selenium Concentrations in Organic Milk: A Systematic Literature Review and Meta- and Redundancy Analyses," *British Journal of Nutrition* 115, no. 6 (2016): 1043–1060, https://doi.org/10.1017/S0007114516000349.

10 Dominika Średnicka-Tober et al., "Composition Differences between Organic and Conventional Meat: A Systematic Literature Review and Meta-Analysis," *British Journal of Nutrition* 115, no. 6 (2016): 994–1011, https://doi.org/10.1017/S0007114515005073.

11 "Recombinant Bovine Growth Hormone," Risk, Prevention, and Screening, American Cancer Society, last modified September 10, 2014, https://www.cancer.org/healthy/cancer-causes/chemicals/recombinant-bovine-growth-hormone.html.

12 Y. H. Chiu et al., "Fruit and Vegetable Intake and Their Pesticide Residues in Relation to Semen Quality among Men from a Fertility Clinic," *Human Reproduction* 30, no. 6 (June 2015): 1346, https://doi.org/10.1093/humrep/dev064.

13 Masoud Neghab et al., "The Effects of Exposure to Pesticides on the Fecundity Status of Farm Workers Resident in a Rural Region of Fars Province, Southern Iran," *Asian Pacific Journal of Tropical Biomedicine* 4, no. 4 (April 2014): 324–328, https://doi.org/10.12980/APJTB.4.2014C586.

14 Ingrid Gerhard et al., "Heavy Metals and Fertility," *Journal of Toxicology and Environmental Health, Part A* 54, no. 8 (1998): 593–611, https://doi.org/10.1080/009841098158638.

15 Prashant Singh et al., "Global Prevalence of Celiac Disease: Systematic Review and Meta-Analysis," *Clinical Gastroenterology and Hepatology* 16, no. 6 (June 2018): 823–836, https://doi.org/10.1016/j.cgh.2017.06.037.

16 Christian Løvold Storhaug, Svein Kjetil Fosse, and Lars T. Fadnes, "Country, Regional, and Global Estimates for Lactose Malabsorption in Adults: A Systematic Review and Meta-Analysis," *The Lancet: Gastroenterology and Hepatology* 2, no. 10 (October 2017): 738–746, https://doi.org/10.1016/s2468-1253(17)30154-1.

17 F. Bolúmar et al., "Caffeine Intake and Delayed Conception: A European Multicenter Study on Infertility and Subfecundity," *American Journal of Epidemiology* 145, no. 4 (February 1997): 324–334, https://doi.org/10.1093/oxfordjournals.aje.a009109.

18 "Fluid Guide," *GrowBaby Health* (blog), April 14, 2022, https://www.growbabyhealth.com/blog/preconceptionpregnancyfluidguide.

19 "How Much Coffee Can I Drink while I'm Pregnant?" Ask ACOG, American College of Obstetricians and Gynecologists, October 2020, https://www.acog.org/womens-health/experts-and-stories/ask-acog/how-much-coffee-can-i-drink-while-pregnant.

20 Rakesh Sharma et al., "Lifestyle Factors and Reproductive Health: Taking Control of Your Fertility," *Reproductive Biology and Endocrinology* 11 (2013): 66, https://doi.org/10.1186/1477-7827-11-66; Zohra S. Lassi et al., "Preconception Care: Caffeine, Smoking, Alcohol, Drugs and Other Environmental Chemical/Radiation Exposure," *Reproductive Health* 11, no. Suppl 3 (2014): S6, https://doi.org/10.1186/1742-4755-11-S3-S6.

21 Brooke V. Rossi et al., "Effect of Alcohol Consumption on In Vitro Fertilization," *Obstetrics and Gynecology* 117, no. 1 (January 2011): 136–142, https://doi.org/10.1097/AOG.0b013e31820090e1.

22 Mohammad Yaser Anwar, Michele Marcus, and Kira C. Taylor, "The Association between Alcohol Intake and Fecundability during Menstrual Cycle Phases," *Human Reproduction* 36, no. 9 (September 2021): 2538–2548, https://doi.org/10.1093/humrep/deab121.

23 Tina Kold Jensen et al., "Habitual Alcohol Consumption Associated with Reduced Semen Quality and Changes in Reproductive Hormones: A Cross-Sectional Study among 1221 Young Danish Men," *BMJ Open* 4, no. 9 (2014): e005462, https://doi.org/10.1136/bmjopen-2014-005462.

24 M. Pourentezari et al., "Additional Deleterious Effects of Alcohol Consumption on Sperm Parameters and DNA Integrity in Diabetic

Mice," *Andrologia* 48, no. 5 (June 2016): 564–569, https://doi.
org/10.1111/and.12481; B. Himabindu, P. Madhu, and P. Sreenivasula
Reddy, "Diabetes and Alcohol: Double Jeopardy with Regard to
Oxidative Toxicity and Sexual Dysfunction in Adult Male Wistar
Rats," *Reproductive Toxicology* 51 (January 2015): 57–63, https://Doi.
Org/10.1016/J.Reprotox.2014.12.010.

25 *GrowBaby Health* (blog), "Fluid Guide."

26 Kara Fitzgerald, *Younger You: Reduce Your Bio Age and Live Longer,
Better* (New York: Hachette Go, 2022), 8.

27 Fitzgerald, *Younger You*, 9–10.

28 J. E. Chavarro et al., "A Prospective Study of Dairy Foods Intake and
Anovulatory Infertility," *Human Reproduction* 22, no. 5 (May 2007):
1340–1347, https://doi.org/10.1093/humrep/dem019.

29 K. Shane Broughton, Jayme Bayes, and Bruce Culver, "High
α-Linolenic Acid and Fish Oil Ingestion Promotes Ovulation to
the Same Extent in Rats," *Nutrition Research* 30, no. 10 (October
2010): 731–738, https://doi.org/10.1016/j.nutres.2010.09.005; Sunni
L. Mumford et al., "Dietary Fat Intake and Reproductive Hormone
Concentrations and Ovulation in Regularly Menstruating Women,"
The American Journal of Clinical Nutrition 103, no. 3 (March 2016):
868–877, https://doi.org/10.3945/ajcn.115.119321.

30 N. F. Boyd et al., "Effects of a Low-Fat High-Carbohydrate Diet on
Plasma Sex Hormones in Premenopausal Women: Results from a
Randomized Controlled Trial," *British Journal of Cancer* 76, no. 1
(1997): 127–135, https://doi.org/10.1038/bjc.1997.348.

31 Surinder Baines, Jennifer Powers, and Wendy J. Brown, "How Does
the Health and Well-Being of Young Australian Vegetarian and
Semi-Vegetarian Women Compare with Non-Vegetarians?" *Public
Health Nutrition* 10, no. 5 (2007): 436–442, https://doi.org/10.1017/
S1368980007217938.

32 Karl M. Pirke et al., "Dieting Influences the Menstrual Cycle:
Vegetarian versus Nonvegetarian Diet," *Fertility and Sterility* 46,
no. 6 (December 1986): 1083–1088, https://doi.org/10.1016/S0015-
0282(16)49884-5.

13. Prenatal Vitamins Are Necessary but Not Sufficient

1 Mark Hyman, "Do You Need Supplements?" *DrHyman* (blog),
accessed March 31, 2023, https://drhyman.com/blog/2015/04/02/do-
you-need-supplements/.

2 Folami Y. Ideraabdullah et al., "Maternal Vitamin D Deficiency and Developmental Origins of Health and Disease (DOHaD)," *Journal of Endocrinology* 241, no. 2 (2019): R65–R80, https://doi.org/10.1530/JOE-18-0541.

3 Ingrid P. C. Krapels et al., "Maternal Dietary B Vitamin Intake, Other Than Folate, and the Association with Orofacial Cleft in the Offspring," *European Journal of Nutrition* 43, no. 1 (2004): 7–14, https://doi.org/10.1007/s00394-004-0433-y; Ingrid P.C. Krapels et al., "*Myo*-Inositol, Glucose and Zinc Status as Risk Factors for Non-Syndromic Cleft Lip with or without Cleft Palate in Offspring: A Case–Control Study," *BJOG* 111, no. 7 (July 2004): 661–668, https://doi.org/10.1111/j.1471-0528.2004.00171.x.

4 E. R. Ellsworth-Bowers and E. J. Corwin, "Nutrition and the Psychoneuroimmunology of Postpartum Depression," *Nutrition Research Reviews* 25, no. 1 (2012): 180–192, https://doi.org/10.1017/S0954422412000091.

5 Nynke van den Broek, "Anaemia and Micronutrient Deficiencies: Reducing Maternal Death and Disability during Pregnancy," *British Medical Bulletin* 67, no. 1 (December 2003): 149–160, https://doi.org/10.1093/bmb/ldg004.

6 Gretchen A. Stevens et al., "Micronutrient Deficiencies among Preschool-Aged Children and Women of Reproductive Age Worldwide: A Pooled Analysis of Individual-Level Data from Population-Representative Surveys," *The Lancet: Global Health* 10, no. 11 (November 2022): E1590–E1599, https://doi.org/10.1016/S2214-109X(22)00367-9.

7 Rebecca J. Schmidt et al., "Association of Maternal Prenatal Vitamin Use with Risk for Autism Spectrum Disorder Recurrence in Young Siblings," *JAMA Psychiatry* 76, no. 4 (2019): 391–398, https://doi.org/10.1001/jamapsychiatry.2018.3901.

8 Nancy L. Morse, "Benefits of Docosahexaenoic Acid, Folic Acid, Vitamin D and Iodine on Foetal and Infant Brain Development and Function following Maternal Supplementation during Pregnancy and Lactation," *Nutrients* 4, no. 7 (2012): 799, https://doi.org/10.3390/nu4070799.

9 I. Romieu et al., "Maternal Fish Intake during Pregnancy and Atopy and Asthma in Infancy," *Clinical and Experimental Allergy* 37, no. 4 (April 2007): 518–525, https://doi.org/10.1111/j.1365-2222.2007.02685.x.

10 "Nutrient Deficiencies May Be at the Root Cause of PCOS," *SpectraCell Laboratories* (blog), January 5, 2023, https://www.

spectracell.com/blog/posts/nutrient-deficiencies-may-be-at-the-root-cause-of-pcos.

11 "The Approach," The Science, ARMRA, accessed March 31, 2023, https://tryarmra.com/pages/the-approach.

12 ARMRA, "The Approach."

13 Vittorio Unfer et al., "Myo-Inositol Effects in Women with PCOS: A Meta-Analysis of Randomized Controlled Trials," *Endocrine Connections* 6, no. 8 (2017): 647–658, https://doi.org/10.1530/EC-17-0243.

14. Move It to Groove It

1 Diana Vaamonde et al., "Physically Active Men Show Better Semen Parameters and Hormone Values Than Sedentary Men," *European Journal of Applied Physiology* 112, no. 9 (2012): 3267–3273, https://doi.org/10.1007/s00421-011-2304-6.

2 Guido Iaccarino et al., "Modulation of Insulin Sensitivity by Exercise Training: Implications for Cardiovascular Prevention," *Journal of Cardiovascular Translational Research* 14, no. 2 (2021): 256–270, https://doi.org/10.1007/s12265-020-10057-w.

3 Audrey Jane Gaskins et al., "Physical Activity and Television Watching in Relation to Semen Quality in Young Men," *British Journal of Sports Medicine* 49, no. 4 (February 2015): 265–270, http://dx.doi.org/10.1136/bjsports-2012-091644.

4 Bin Sun et al., "Physical Activity and Sedentary Time in Relation to Semen Quality in Healthy Men Screened as Potential Sperm Donors," *Human Reproduction* 34, no. 12 (December 2019): 2330–2339, https://doi.org/10.1093/humrep/dez226.

5 https://pronatalfitness.com/.

6 "Moving Guide," *GrowBaby Health* (blog), March 11, 2019, https://www.growbabyhealth.com/blog/moving-guide.

7 Edward R. Laskowski, "What Are the Risks or Sitting Too Much?" Adult Health, Healthy Lifestyle, Mayo Clinic, July 13, 2022, https://www.mayoclinic.org/healthy-lifestyle/adult-health/expert-answers/sitting/faq-20058005.

8 Manuel Dote-Montero et al., "Acute Effect of HIIT on Testosterone and Cortisol Levels in Healthy Individuals: A Systematic Review and Meta-Analysis," *Scandinavian Journal of Medicine and Science in Sports* 31, no. 9 (September 2021): 1722–1744, https://doi.org/10.1111/sms.13999.

9   Brooke V. Rossi, Mary Abusief, and Stacey A. Missmer, "Modifiable
    Risk Factors and Infertility: What Are the Connections?" *American
    Journal of Lifestyle Medicine* 10, no. 4 (2016): 226–227, https://doi.
    org/10.1177/1559827614558020.
10 Rossi, Abusief, and Missmer, "Modifiable Risk Factors," 226;
    Chavarro et al., "Diet and Lifestyle."
11 Committee on Obstetric Practice, American Society for
    Reproductive Medicine, "ACOG Committee Opinion No. 804:
    Physical Activity and Exercise during Pregnancy and the
    Postpartum Period," *Obstetrics & Gynecology* 135, no. 4 (April 2020):
    e182, https://doi.org/10.1097/AOG.0000000000003772.
12 Jorge E. Chavarro et al., "Diet and Lifestyle in the Prevention of
    Ovulatory Disorder Infertility," *Obstetrics and Gynecology* 110,
    no. 5 (November 2007): 1053–1054, https://doi.org/10.1097/01.
    aog.0000287293.25465.e1.

15. Get Your Mental Game in Order

1   Mary E. Coussons-Read, "Effects of Prenatal Stress on Pregnancy
    and Human Development: Mechanisms and Pathways,"
    Obstetric Medicine 6, no. 2 (June 2013): 52–57, https://doi.
    org/10.1177/1753495X12473751.
2   Joanna Jurewicz et al., "Wpływ stresu aawodowego na jakość nasienia,"
    [The effect of stress on the semen quality], *Medycyna Pracy* 61, no. 6
    (2010): 607–613, https://pubmed.ncbi.nlm.nih.gov/21452563/.
3   U.S. Centers for Disease Control and Prevention, "1 in 3 Adults
    Don't Get Enough Sleep," news release, February 18, 2016, https://
    www.cdc.gov/media/releases/2016/p0215-enough-sleep.html; Eric
    Suni, "What Causes Insomnia?" Sleep Foundation, last modified
    March 3, 2023, https://www.sleepfoundation.org/insomnia.
4   Kelly McGonigal, *The Upside of Stress: Why Stress Is Good for You,
    and How to Get Good at It* (New York: Avery, 2015), 66, 14.
5   Emily Fletcher, "This One Thing Will Keep You Resilient in the Face
    of Stress & Anxiety," *Ziva* (blog), accessed March 31, 2023, https://
    zivameditation.com/blog/this-one-thing-will-keep-you-resilient-in-
    the-face-of-stress-anxiety/.
6   Nick Ortner, *The Tapping Solution: A Revolutionary System for
    Stress-Free Living* (Carlsbad, CA: Hay House, 2013), 6.
7   Patrick L. Hill, Mathias Allemand, and Brent W. Roberts,
    "Examining the Pathways between Gratitude and Self-Rated

Physical Health across Adulthood," *Personality and Individual Differences* 54, no. 1 (January 2013): 92–96, https://doi.org/10.1016/j.paid.2012.08.011.

16. *The Real Sex Ed*

1   Allen J. Wilcox, Clarice R. Weinberg, and Donna D. Baird, "Timing of Sexual Intercourse in Relation to Ovulation—Effects on the Probability of Conception, Survival of the Pregnancy, and Sex of the Baby," *The New England Journal of Medicine* 333, no. 23 (December 7, 1995): 1517–1521, https://doi.org/10.1056/NEJM199512073332301.

2   *The Great Sperm Race*, directed by Julian Jones (London: ITV Global, 2009).

3   *Great Sperm Race*.

4   *Great Sperm Race*.

5   Josleen Wilson, *The Pre-Pregnancy Planner* (Garden City, NY: Doubleday & Company, 1986), 65.

6   Nicholas Pound et al., "Duration of Sexual Arousal Predicts Semen Parameters for Masturbatory Ejaculates," *Physiology and Behavior* 76, no. 4–5 (August 2002): 685–689, https://doi.org/10.1016/S0031-9384(02)00803-X.

ACKNOWLEDGMENTS

My mother—for epitomizing what unconditional love looks like every single day of my life. No words could ever express how grateful I am to be your daughter. Thank you for being there for every step and turn of the Poplin journey—reading all my emails, problem solving messaging and positioning, printing posters, creating boxes, the list goes on. I couldn't have done it without you.

My father—for teaching me the CCD (confidence, commitment, and discipline) principle and for being an example of it in your own life, for supporting me even when you had no idea where I was headed, and for always holding me to high standards. You are the quiet but strong voice inside that keeps me going.

My partner—for sharing every bit of life alongside me; for being my anchor, my source of stability, my grounding as I undertook the wild journey of entrepreneurship and authorship; for giving me the space to try things and to fail; for being brilliant; for challenging my thinking; and for always sharing real talk, not just telling me what I wanted to hear. I am stronger and better because of you and am grateful beyond words for what's been and what's to come.

My sister, Christina—for letting me see motherhood through your eyes, for making me an auntie, for showing me what it means to persevere, for putting up with all of my idiosyncrasies.

My sister, Cassandra—for cheering me on; for cheering me up; for telling me like it is; for being a beta tester, a graphic designer, a copywriter, and so many more roles in the early days; for never losing faith in me.

My brother-in-law, Kennon—for being willing to nerd out with me on all things biohacking and for being an outspoken supporter and publicist from day one.

My nephews, Alexander and Anthony—you are my ultimate inspiration; you make me want to be better and do better. I am so incredibly proud to be your auntie, and I cannot wait to see what amazing things you do in this world.

My best friend, Sarah—for being there through it all; for following me, then for leading the way; for your unwavering support; for being the awe-inspiring person, friend, and entrepreneur that you are. I am so lucky to have you in my orbit.

My Friday Founders group (Amy, Emily, Narmeen)— for being a consistent source of inspiration and support; for walking alongside me on this winding entrepreneurial journey; for practically helping me with so many things along the way, big and small alike.

So many other friends who were early supporters and have provided advice and perspective along the way.

Kristy Goodman—for trusting me to continue the work that you so beautifully started.

My team (Jennifer D'Aponte, Gretchen DePalma, Joane de Paz, and our extended team)—thank you for making work fun and for doing all that you do to help amplify the message of pre-pregnancy wellness through Poplin. Thank you to those that have contributed along the way to other pieces of the Poplin journey—Krešimir Bojčić, Mateo Vukušić, Marko Matotan, Filip Piškur, Ela Prižmić Šivak, Marko Razum and extended team, Erik Ibarra, Steven Gonzalez, Paul Barron and team, Taryn Laeben Jones, Kate O'Connor, Joyce Schmulson, Jackson Corey and team, Emily Taylor, Martha Anderson, our lab partners and collaborators—and many more.

My functional medicine teachers (Dr. Kara Fitzgerald, Dr. Gary Goldman, Dana James, Lara Zakaria, Romilly Hodges)—thank you for shepherding me into the world of functional medicine and for teaching me its power to heal. It opened me to new possibilities and planted the seed for the book you hold in your hands now.

Those who came before me and laid the groundwork and whose work I took inspiration from. Those who published books and studies that have furthered the interests of functional medicine, integrative fertility, and preconception care. There are too many to list, but a few that stand out: Aimee Raupp, Dr. Marc Sklar, Christa Orecchio, Dr. Jolene Brighten, Rebecca Fett, Jill Blakeway, Nim Barnes, Dr. Jorge Chavarro and Dr. Walter Willett, Robert Cefalo and Merry-K. Moos, Dr. Mark Hyman, Dr. Aviva Romm, Nicole Jardim, Dave Asprey and Dr. Lana Asprey, Dr. Leslie Stone and Emily Rydbom, Chris Kresser, Jessica Drummond.

My clients—for sharing their stories with me, for trusting me, for letting me share a small piece of their journey.

Poplin's investors—for believing in me and in the mission of Poplin to make preconception care mainstream.

The team at Scribe—for teaching me how to write a book and then helping me make it happen.

ABOUT THE AUTHOR

Alexandria DeVito, MS, CNS, is a functional nutritionist who specializes in fertility and preconception health. She is the founder of Poplin, the first pre-pregnancy wellness company. Poplin empowers conceiving couples to take control of their pre-pregnancy journey with a step-by-step preparation process, starting with the most comprehensive pre-pregnancy wellness lab testing available on the market.

Prior to founding Poplin, Alexandria spent a decade in the corporate world, including management consulting at McKinsey & Company and investment banking at Bank of America Merrill Lynch. Alexandria holds dual master's degrees—a Master of Business Administration from Harvard Business School and a Master of Science in Human Nutrition from the University of Bridgeport. Additionally, she has undergone extensive training as a doula, yoga teacher, personal trainer, and eating psychology coach, all of which inform her approach to pre-pregnancy wellness. Alexandria is also an Institute for Functional Medicine Certified Practitioner, one of only two thousand in the world.

Made in United States
North Haven, CT
16 February 2024

48822622R00214